Advanced Examination Techniques in Orthopaedics

For
Becky, Lucy, Rosie, Molly
&
Desmond

Advanced Examination Techniques in Orthopaedics

Edited by

Nick Harris FRCS(Tr and Orth)

Assistant Editor

David Stanley BSc(Hons) FRCS

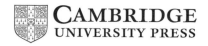
CAMBRIDGE
UNIVERSITY PRESS

CAMBRIDGE UNIVERSITY PRESS
Cambridge, New York, Melbourne, Madrid, Cape Town, Singapore, São Paulo, Delhi

Cambridge University Press
The Edinburgh Building, Cambridge CB2 8RU, UK

Published in the United States of America by Cambridge University Press, New York

www.cambridge.org
Information on this title: www.cambridge.org/9780521862417

First published 2003
Reprinted by Cambridge University Press 2005
Third printing 2008

Printed in the United Kingdom at the University Press, Cambridge

A catalogue record for this publication is available from the British Library

ISBN 978-0-521-86241-7 hardback

Contents

Contributors

Mr L C Bainbridge FRCS
Derby Royal Infirmary
Derby

Mr M J Bell FRCS
Sheffield Children's Hospital, Western Bank,
Sheffield

Mr D R Bickerstaff MD FRCS
Sheffield Centre for Sports Medicine
Sheffield

Mr S H Bostock FRCS(Tr and Orth)
Northern General Hospital
Sheffield

Mr P Calvert MA FRCS
St George's Hospital
London

Mr N Chiverton FRCS(Tr and Orth)
Northern General Hospital
Sheffield

Professor R A Dickson MA ChM FRCS DSc
Clinical Sciences Building, St James's Hospital
Leeds

Mr James Fernandez FRCS(Tr and Orth)
Sheffield Children's Hospital, Western Bank,
Sheffield

Mr C J M Getty MA FRCS
Northern General Hospital
Sheffield

Mr N J Harris FRCS(Tr and Orth)
Leeds General Infirmary
Leeds

Mr R E Page ChM FRCS
Northern General Hospital
Sheffield

Mr T W D Smith FRCS, FRCS(Ed)
Northern General Hospital
Sheffield

Mr J Srinivasan
Derby Royal Infirmary
Derby

Mr D Stanley BSc(Hons) FRCS
Northern General Hospital
Sheffield

Mr M M Stephens MSc(Bioeng), FRCSI
Foot Clinics, Children's Hospital, Temple Street
Dublin 1, Ireland

Mr I G Stockley MD FRCS
Northern General Hospital
Sheffield

Preface

The original concept for the book arose when I was preparing for my FRCS(Tr and Orth) Exam. I found it difficult to quickly revise special tests on clinical examination. If you wanted to look at tests for postero-lateral rotatory instability of the knee you had to get a specialist text on knee surgery. Similarly if you wanted to review tests for rotator cuff tear of the the shoulder you had to get a specialist text on shoulder surgery. Those existing books that covered clinical examination seemed too basic for what I needed. They were aimed mainly at medical students. The aim therefore was to compile a book looking at advanced examination techniques in orthopaedics. Each chapter has been written by an expert or under the supervision of an expert in that area. Rather than produce long lists of different clinical tests we asked the contributors to describe which tests they found most useful in their day to day practice. The foundation for a good clinical examination will always be inspection, palpatation and movement. If this can be followed up with directed specific tests it is often possible to make an accurate diagnosis without the need for other expensive investigations.

As well as being of value to the Orthopaedic Registrar approaching the FRCS(Tr and Orth) Exam the book will also be of interest to physiotherapists, sports physicians, rheumatologists and G.P.'s.

N.H.
Leeds
September 2002

Foreword

With the meteoric increase in reliance on advanced technology for diagnosis and treatment, a return to the basics is a careful physical examination. This work represents a very interesting approach to the physical examination and is true to its title of *Advanced Examination Techniques*. This effort would certainly support the mantra "When in doubt, examine the patient." This orientation has never been more true than today, and this textbook goes a long way in aiding the orthopedic surgeon along this path.

Yet, one might question the need for a text such as this given the existence of other such works. The value of this contribution is the thorough and comprehensive nature of the text and the clarity of photographs and ease of reference. Many of the examinations and diagnoses are not readily available in previous works. The consistent format is certainly user-friendly and allows a valuable and updated compendium of physical signs as well as the details of the examination. It goes without saying the attractiveness in no small measure is also enhanced by the subjects in which the examinations are being demonstrated.

The authors have realized the goals stated in the preface, and I anticipate that the reader will find this not only a valuable and interesting reference source, but also an enjoyable one.

Bernard F. Morrey, M.D.
The Mayo Clinic
Rochester, Minnesota
USA

Acknowledgements

There are many people I need to thank who helped with the production of this book. Dave Stanley gave me the initial encouragement to approach the publishers with the idea in the first place. Greenwich Medical Media have been very patient with my attempts to meet some of the deadlines promised. Gavin Smith in particular has been very flexible in the construction of the book. Howmedica and Chris Lloyd provided funds for the models and photographer. Yvonne Paul Management who provided the models and George Richardson the photographer worked hard to ensure we got all the illustrations we needed in the one shoot. Jade and Leilani were truly professional models.

My greatest thanks go to the contrubutors all of whom have made family and professional sacrifices to ensure we received their relevant chapters on time. I am also especially grateful for the support and encouragement I have received throughout my training from Tom Smith, Mike Bell and Ian Stockley.

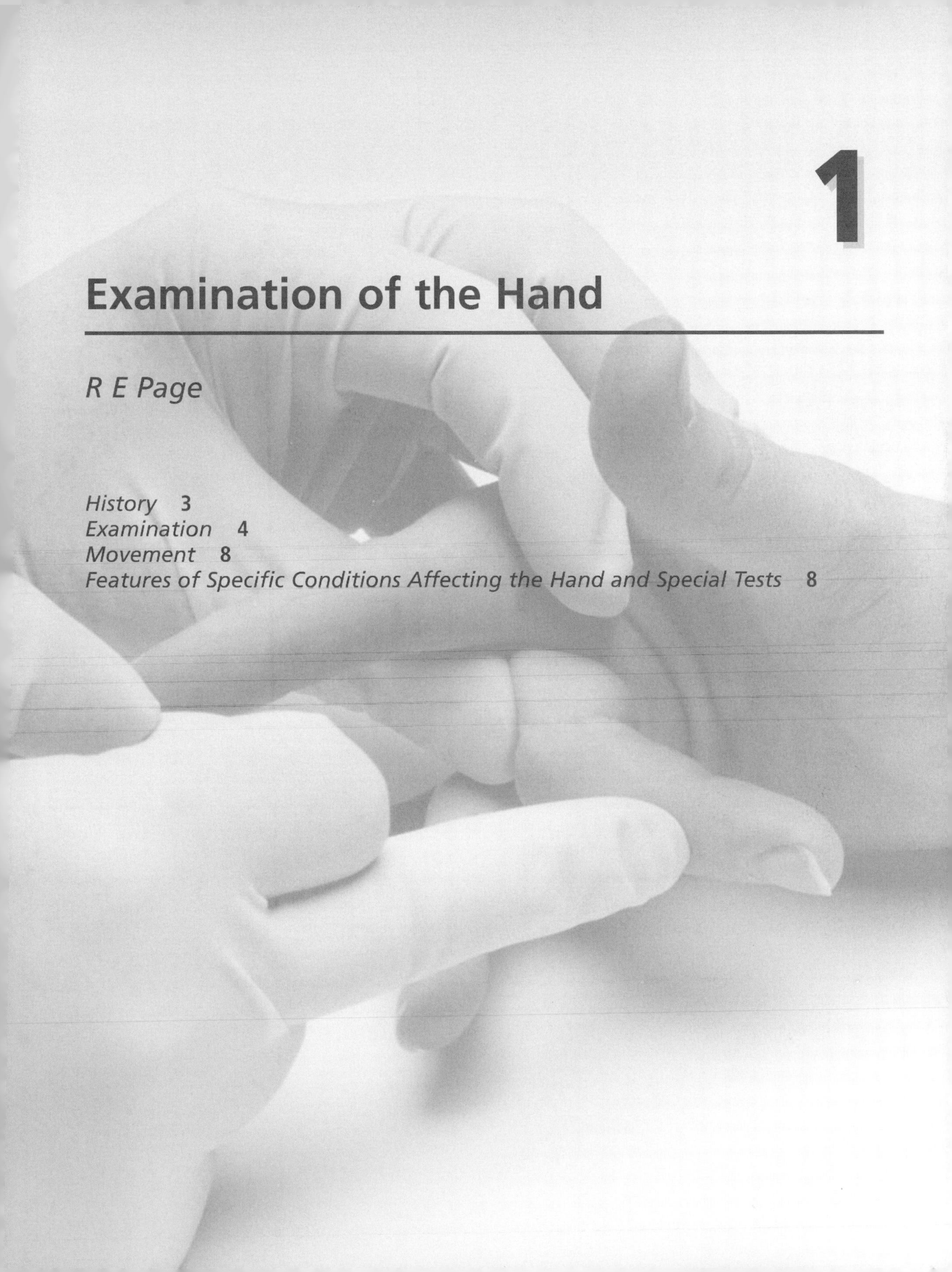

Examination of the Hand

R E Page

1

History

General

Establish important details such as age, dominance, occupation, hobbies, social status, nature of the injury (involvement with compensation), general health including pre-existing conditions such as diabetes, gout, arthritis, collagen disease (SLE, Lupus), drugs and allergies. Allow the patient to describe the symptoms, which will be among those listed below. There are many pathological conditions affecting the hand but it is usually possible to arrive at a provisional diagnosis early in the consultation at which point specific questions pertinent to the condition can commence.

Specific symptoms

Pain

This is a very common presenting complaint as it is a feature of infection, inflammation, arthritis, trauma and nerve compression. Unrelenting night pain causing loss of sleep is strongly suggestive of deep seated infection. Pain on movement will focus attention on joints or tendons. Pain associated with altered sensation suggests nerve entrapment.

Swelling

Swelling may be localised or generalised. The loose tissues on the dorsum of the hand allow for a greater degree of swelling than the palmar aspect where the skin is more tightly anchored to underlying structures (**Figure 1**).

Weakness

If this symptom is associated with pain it may be due to tendon or joint disease rather than neuromuscular disorders.

Numbness

Patients often have great difficulty in accurately outlining the distribution of this symptom. The lack of an anatomically compatible description does not invalidate the complaint.

Deformity

This will be obvious in trauma and cases suffering the various forms of arthritis.

Instability

Joint instability accompanies ligamentous disruption following trauma as in gamekeeper's thumb,

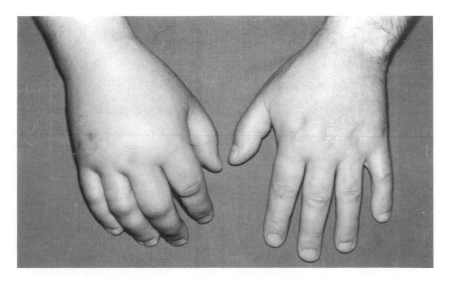

Figure 1 Swelling of loose dorsal tissues of the right hand as a result of a palmar space infection.

but may arise as a feature of osteo or rheumatoid arthritis where ligaments are destroyed or attenuated by the disease process. Occasionally non-union of a fracture may cause instability.

Snapping tendons

On moving the hand into flexion the patient may notice snapping of the extensor tendons over the MCP joints. It is usually due to disruption of the juncture tendons or sagittal bands.

Stiffness

This symptom is usually associated with arthritic change but will also be encountered after trauma and may persist in those patients suffering with post-traumatic sympathetic dystrophy. (see later)

Loss of dexterity

Loss of manipulative skills may be due to a number of different causes but deranged activity of the intrinsic muscles should always be considered.

Cold intolerance

Most patients after trauma or surgery will encounter cold intolerance for a number of years. It is manifested as an aching discomfort associated with capillary vascular changes resulting in a bluish, purple discolouration of the skin. Stiffness will also trouble the patient.

Congenital

It is important to ask about a family history and enquire about illnesses or drug therapy during pregnancy.

Examination

The basic equipment required for any hand examination should include a pin wheel, dividers for 2PD, Jamar & Pinch dynamometer and a goniometer.

General

The whole of the upper limb should be exposed on both sides to allow for comparison then LOOK, FEEL, MOVE. Start with the dorsal aspect of the hand including the nails, then proceed to the volar side.

Posture

At rest there will be a moderate degree of dorsi flexion of the wrist and some ulnar deviation. Flexion of the MCP and PIP joints increases from the index to the little fingers. The thumb will be in a slightly abducted position with the pulp lying close to the DIP joint of the index. Disease processes will alter this natural posture particularly nerve deficits, for example the "main en griffe" deformity in combined high ulnar and median nerve lesions.

Tremor

This may suggest anxiety or thyrotoxicosis when fine or a benign essential tremor or Parkinson's disease when coarse. Beware the hysterical tremor usually coarse in type, often seen on examining grip strength in a patient set on compensation.

Size

It is useful to observe the size of the hands as it has been suggested that large thick set hands respond more slowly to treatment than small thin hands. When hands appear disproportionately large then consider acromegaly.

Swelling

Localised swelling with redness and heat will indicate an active infective or inflammatory condition. Ganglia from any source of synovium (joint or tendon), are by far the most common cause of cystic swellings, Giant cell tumours of tendon sheath are the commonest cause of isolated solid swellings. Swelling of the whole hand is more easily detected dorsally and may be quite firm as in lymphoedema or Secretan's disease.[1] (Factitious trauma to the dorsum of the hand)

Colour

Vascular lesions will be apparent as localised changes in skin colour. Purple-blue discolouration of the whole hand in association with pain and swelling would indicate post-traumatic sympathetic dystrophy. Persistent bruising in the vicinity of ligaments is strongly suggestive of rupture. Vascular integrity of the hand can be assessed using the Allen's test. This can be performed for the whole hand or the individual digits, which is especially indicated in patients undergoing revision surgery for Dupytren's disease.

Nails

A wide range of medical conditions affect the nails for example, clubbing, splinter haemorrhages, beware the subungual melanoma. Mucus cysts will cause grooving of the nail. Non-traumatic destruction of the nail is usually due to tumour. Subungual glomus tumours are extremely painful when the nail is knocked and usually appear as a localised blue-purple blush in the sterile matrix.

Creases

Where joints are immobile skin creases are absent (**Figure 2**).

Deformity

Congenital abnormalities, arthritis and trauma are the common causes.

Muscle wasting

This is most likely to be detected in the ulnar innervated 1st dorsal interosseous, in the 1st web space or in the median innervated abductor pollicis brevis in the thenar eminence.

Sensation

Light touch should be tested in the median, ulnar and radial nerve distributions. Absent sweating detected by the biro test or skin conductance measurements is a sign of denervation. In the biro test the body of the pen runs smoothly along a dry denervated digit whereas it drags when it is run along a moist normally innervated finger. The water immersion test can be useful in children. After 5-10 minutes in warm water innervated finger pulps pucker, denervated pulps remain smooth.

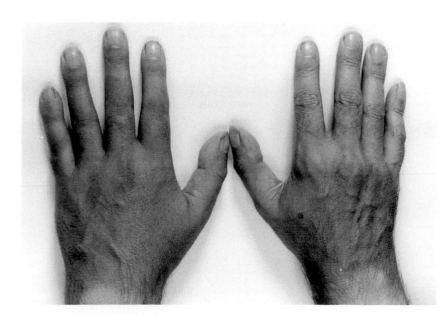

Figure 2 As a result of end-stage post traumatic sympathetic dystrophy this patient has completely stiff PIP and DIP joints on the left hand. Note the lack of skin creasing over the joints.

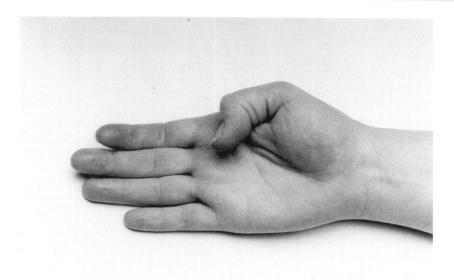

Figure 3 (a) Flexion*

*Note the Linburg Comstock sign where FPL action also initiates FDP flexion in the index finger by means of an anomalous communicating tendon.

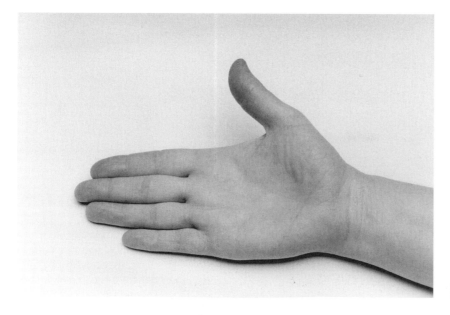

Figure 3 (b) Extension

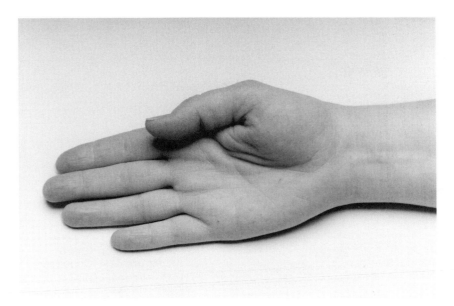

Figure 3 (c) Adduction

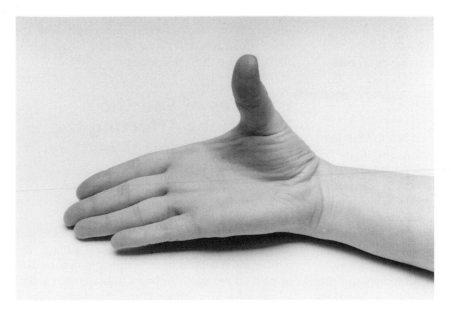

Figure 3 (d) Abduction

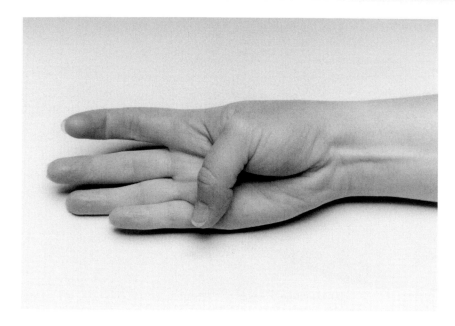

Figure 3 (e) Opposition

Crepitus

Over tendons this will suggest tenosynovitis and over joints arthritic change.

Thrill

This may be detected in a high flow vascular malformation or in relation to an arterio-venous fistula.

Movement

The MCP joints will move from 0-90°, the PIP joint 0-110° and the DIP joint 0-90°. As the digits flex they follow an equi angular spiral (progressive spiral as described by Fibonacci). As a fist is formed the 4th and 5th CMC joints flex dropping the level of the metacarpal heads. Flexion and extension movements alone will take place at the PIP and DIP joints. The MCP joints allow abduction and adduction of the fingers, with the point of reference along the line of the middle finger. Movements of the thumb are described as abduction, adduction,

extension, flexion and opposition (**Figure 3**). Active and passive ranges of movements should be elicited. Strength of various movements can be assessed using the MRC scale (**Figure 4**) or alternatively the composite movements of grip can be measured using a Jamar dynamometer and pinch with the pinch dynamometer. Joint stability is tested by stressing the collateral ligaments.

Features of Specific Conditions Affecting the Hand and Special Tests

Flexor tendon injury

History

Any laceration on the volar aspect of the hand may partially or completely divide a flexor tendon. The patient will complain of an inability to flex the digit or pain on flexion. Numbness indicates that a digital nerve has been damaged and this is often associ-

MRC Muscle Power

M0 – No movement

M1 = Flicker of movement

M2 = Movement with gravity excluded

M3 = Movement against gravity but not against examiners resistance

M4 = Less then normal power (poor fair moderate)

M5 = Full power

Figure 4 MRC Muscle Power.

ated with partial tendon injury. In competitive sports a shirt pulling injury may result in rupture of the FDP tendon from the distal phalanx usually involving the ring finger. The patient may complain not only of an inability to flex the DIP joint but also some fullness in the palm due to retraction of the FDP (Leddy classification[2]; **Figure 5**).

Examination

Record the zone of injury I-V. The integrity of each tendon must be established. Division of both tendons to a single digit will result in the pointing sign (**Figure 6**). The FPL, FCR, FCU, FDS and FDP tendon to the index all have separate muscle bellies. The FDP tendons to the middle, ring and little fingers share the same muscle belly (quadriga affect). Thus any block to the profundus flexion action in one of the ulnar 3 digits will tend to prevent the other 2 from flexing. This phenomenon can be used to separate out the sublimis action across the PIP joint and the profundus action across the DIP joint. (**Figures** 7 and 8). Tenderness on palpation along the flexor aspect of the digit may suggest the possibility of a partially divided tendon. When tendon

movement against resistance causes pain then there may be a partial division. The sublimis tendons to the little fingers are frequently hypo-plastic and both sides should be tested.

Trigger finger / trigger thumb

History

In the neonate triggering usually involves the thumb and will be noticed as a fixed flexion deformity of the IP joint. Adults complain of pain and tenderness at the base of involved digits and a tendency for the finger to catch as the PIP joint is extended. Occasionally the finger may lock in flexion. Diabetic and rheumatoid patients are more prone to this condition.

Examination

In the child the flexion deformity of the IP joint of the thumb can sometimes be passively corrected and there is often a palpable nodule at the level of the A1 pulley. In trigger finger tenderness and occasionally crepitus is apparent at the A1

Leddy Classification of FDP Rupture

Type I – Avulsed FDP retracts into palm

Type II – Tendon retracts to PIP joint level

Type III – A large bony fragment held in the distal pulley

system. Lateral x-ray shows bony fragment just

proximal to DIP joint

Figure 5 Leddy Classification of FDP Rupture.

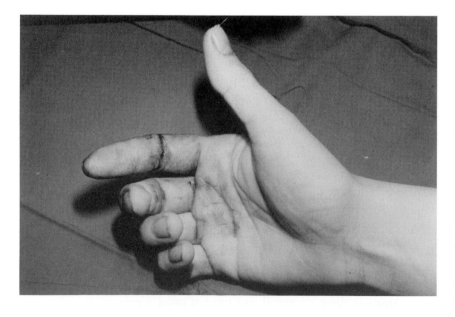

Figure 6 Both flexor tendons of the index have been divided in Zone 2 resulting in the 'Pointing' sign.

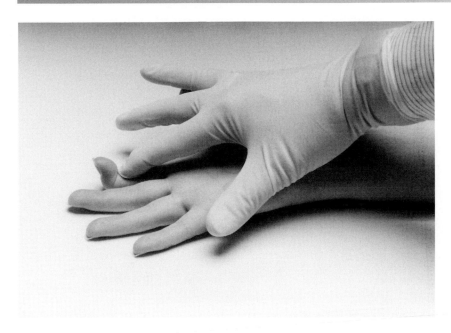

Figure 7 Examination of the FDP tendon to the index.

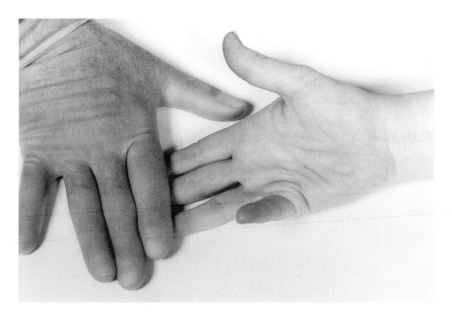

Figure 8 (a) Examination of the sublimus tendons. Note the lack of PIP joint flexion in the little finger indicative of a hypoplastic FDS tendon.

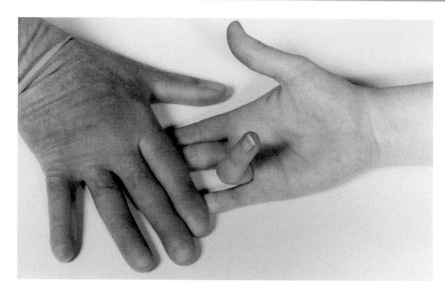

Figure 8 (b)

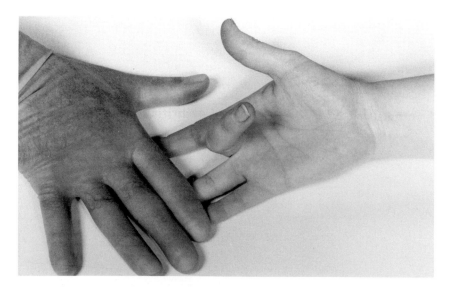

Figure 8 (c)

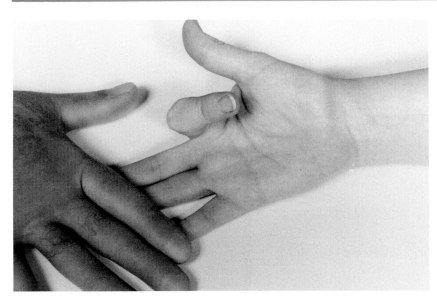

Figure 8 (d)

pulley and often a mobile nodule on the flexor tendons can be detected. In the advanced condition the finger will lock in flexion and on active extension remain flexed before suddenly snapping straight. Rarely triggering can take place more distally as the FDP passes through the sublimis chiasma. Tenderness is then located over the volar aspect of the PIP joint.

Osteoarthritis

History

This can affect any joint in the hand after trauma or infection but commonly involves the DIP and 1st CMC joints. With DIP joint involvement the patient will complain of pain, loss of movement and deformity. When the 1st CMC joint is involved, commonly in middle-aged women, pain at the base of the thumb associated with deformity and loss of pinch strength are common symptoms.

Examination

In arthritis of the DIP joints assessment of the range of movement and stability should be made.

Osteophytes result in Heberden's nodes. Prominent osteophytes arising at the PIP joint are much less common and result in Bouchard's nodes. In 1st CMC joint osteoarthritis, the grind test will be positive, this involves rotating the base of the 1st metacarpal against the trapezium. A positive test results in pain and crepitus. As the disease progresses an adduction deformity of the 1st metacarpal develops associated with secondary hyperextension of the MCP joint (**Figure 9**).

Rheumatoid arthritis

It is important to establish the degree of disability and functional loss. Deformity does not necessarily correlate closely with loss of function (**Figure 10**). In those cases where surgery may be appropriate the patient's drug therapy must be considered as immunosupressives, penicillamine and steroids will have an adverse affect on healing. The state of the patient's cervical spine and temperomandibular joints will be of interest to the anaesthetist. A quick assessment of the shoulder, elbow and wrist should be undertaken as these should receive surgical priority.

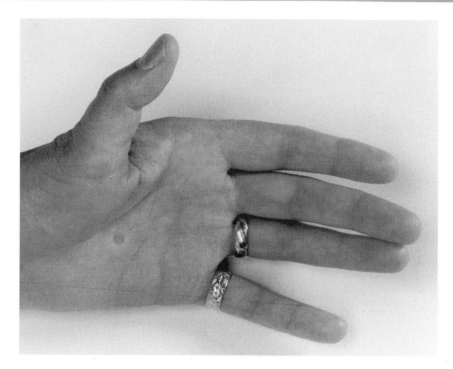

Figure 9 Osteoarthritis of the 1st CMC joint has resulted in subluxation of the joint causing a prominence at the base of the thumb. The 1st metacarpal has become adducted. Secondary hyperextension of the MCP joint allows the thumb to move out of the palm.

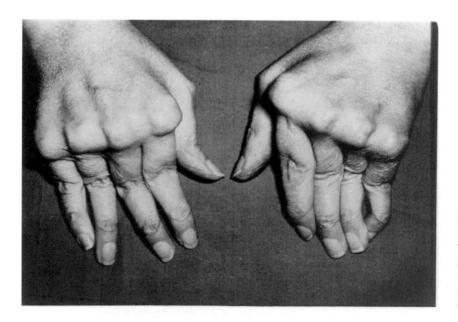

Figure 10 Advanced rheumatoid arthritis with fixed subluxation; note the 2nd-5th MCP joints and ulnar drift on the left side. Multiple swan neck deformities.

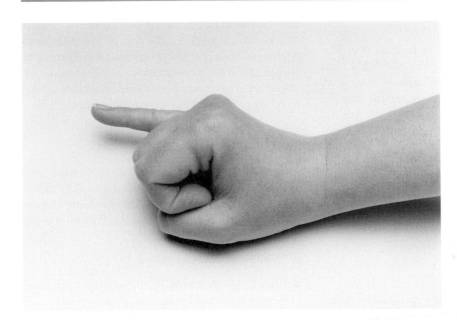

Figure 11 EDQ sign. The little finger is fully extended at the MCP joint indicating an intact EDQ.

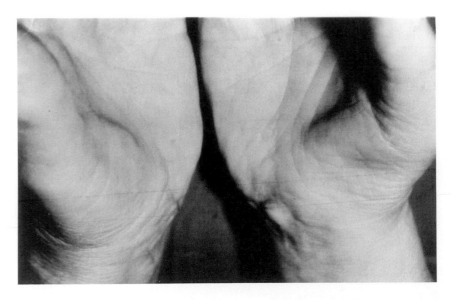

Figure 12 Wasting of the APB in chronic carpal tunnel syndrome.

Flexor synovitis

The patient will complain of a fullness over the volar aspect of the wrist or along the flexor tendon sheaths. Stiffness and a reduced range of flexion are common complaints. Crepitus may be palpable at the wrist or at the level of the A1 pulley, which is best elicited by placing the examining finger transversely across the palm at the level of the A1 pulleys as the patient flexes. In advanced disease, triggering can be troublesome and attrition tendon rupture may occur due to synovial infiltration or wear over bone edges. e.g. FPL round a scaphoid osteophyte (Mannerfelt Lesion.[3])

MCP joints

It is important to establish the active and passive range of movement of the MCP joints together with the degree of subluxation and ulnar drift. Flexor and extensor tendons should be carefully assessed. The EDQ sign (**Figure 11**) will be helpful in detecting rupture of the EDQ which frequently precedes little and ring finger EDC ruptures (Vaughan Jackson lesion[4]) and EPL may rupture over Lister's tubercle. Flexor synovitis may cause carpal tunnel syndrome and there may be wasting of abductor pollicis brevis (**Figure 12**). Where full passive correction of the MCP joints is possible, then soft tissue correction alone may be sufficient. Careful assessment of the PIP joints is also important, as poor stiff immobile joints will detract from the results of MCP joint replacement.

Swan-neck deformity

A swan-neck deformity will result when volar joint structures are weakened by synovitis and the deformity will be promoted by tendon imbalance (**Figure 13**). Nalebuff has described a classification for this deformity:[5]

- **Type I** – all joints mobile
- **Type II** – with the MCP joint extended PIP joint flexion is limited because of ulnar intrinsic tightness. This can be assessed using the Finichietto-Bunnell test (**Figure 14**)
- **Type III** – limited PIP joint flexion in all positions of the MCP joint with good x-ray appearance
- **Type IV** – stiff PIP joints with articular disruption

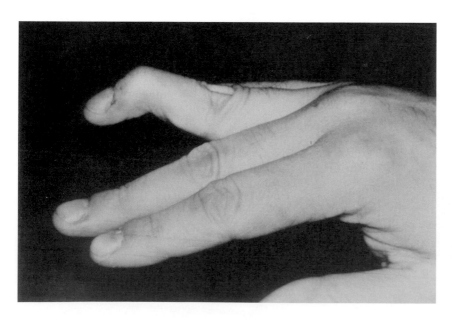

Figure 13 Swan neck deformity. Note the prominent lateral slips.

This classification correlates closely with surgical treatment options.

Boutonniere deformity

Synovial proliferation within the dorsal aspect of the PIP will weaken dorsal structures and result in the Boutonniere deformity (**Figure 15**). As the central slip stretches the 2 lateral bands displace in a volar direction producing flexion of the PIP joint and extension of the DIP joint. The deformity has been classified by Nalebuff.[6]

■ **Stage 1 – mild Boutonniere deformity**

☐ Where there is a slight extensor lag at the PIP joint which can be easily passively corrected but results in limited DIP joint flexion.

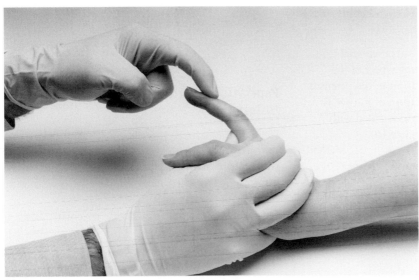

(a)

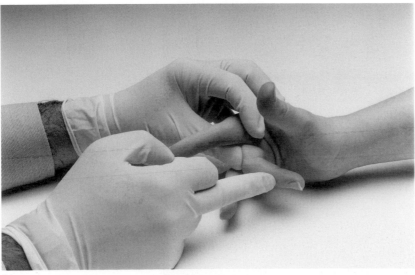

(b)

Figure 14 The Finichietto-Bunnell Test for intrinsic tightness. (a) With the MCP joint passively extended the intrinsic muscle is stretched. If it is tight the PIP joint will be extended and resist passive flexion. (b) With the MCP joint flexed the tight intrinsic will be relaxed and allow passive flexion. By moving the MCP joint from side to side the radial and ulnar intrinsics can be separately assessed.

- **Stage 2 – moderate Boutonniere deformity**
  - ☐ The PIP joint is flexed to 30-40 degrees. On passive extension the shortened lateral slips prevent DIP joint flexion.

- **Stage 3 – severe Boutonniere deformity**
  - ☐ There is no passive extension of the flexed PIP joint and frequently the joint surfaces are destroyed.

Deformities of the thumb

The 4 types originally described by Nalebuff [7] have now been extended to 5.

- **Type 1** – Boutonniere deformity. Synovial proliferation within the dorsal aspect of the MCP joint results in attenuation of the extensor apparatus and some subluxation of the MCP joint which flexes and this is associated with extension of the IP joint (**Figure 16**).

- **Type II** – MCP joint flexion and IP joint hyperextension coupled with subluxation/dislocation of the 1st CMC joint.

- **Type III** – Swan Neck. Involvement of the 1st CMC joint results in an adducted 1st metacarpal with secondary hyperextension of the MCP joint and flexion of the IP joint.

- **Type IV** – The 1st metacarpal is adducted and there is laxity of the ulnar collateral ligament of the MCP joint.

- **Type V** – the volar plate of the MCP joint stretches resulting in hyperextension and there is flexion of the IP joint. There is no adduction deformity of the 1st metacarpal.

Psoriatic arthritis
History

7% of patients with psoriasis will suffer inflammatory arthritis. Some will notice polyarthritis as in rheumatoid arthritis and nearly all patients suffering with psoriatic arthritis will have peripheral joint involvement.

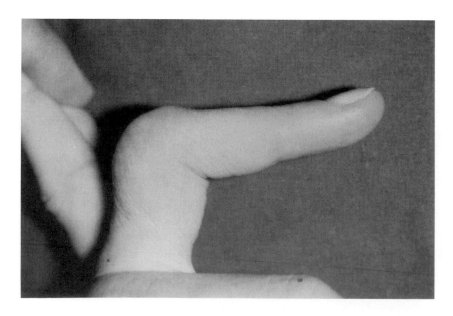

Figure 15 Boutonniere deformity with synovial proliferation in the dorsal aspect of the PIP joint.

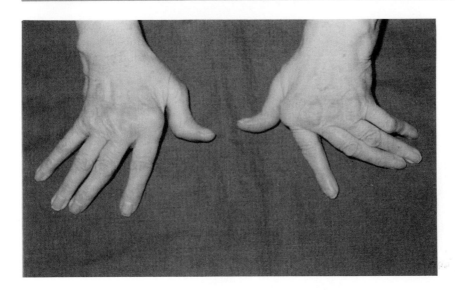

Figure 16 Type I Boutonniere deformities of the thumb.

Examination

In contrast to rheumatoid arthritis, the MCP joints may have extension contractures, pitting of the nails will be obvious (**Figure 17**). Flexion or extension contractures of the PIP joints are commonly encountered. In its severest form arthritis mutilans there is gross skeletal destruction leading to collapsed flail digits (**Figure 18**).

Dupuytren's contracture

History

Ask about the feet as the condition frequently affects the plantar aponeurosis. Typically patients will describe a palmar nodule progressing to a band associated with a fixed flexion deformity of the PIP or MCP joint of the ring or little fingers. There may be a positive history of diabetes, epilepsy, hepatic cirrhosis or AIDS. The index and middle fingers as well as the thumb may be involved. Pain is not a feature of this condition but may occur occasionally on firmly gripping an object in the palm, when nodules can compress the common digital nerves. In recurrent cases make a careful note of those digits that have been the site of previous surgery.

Examination

The extent of the flexion contractures should be noted and these can be recorded with a paperclip-o-gram (a paperclip is bent to lie on the dorsal aspect of the affected digit reflecting the degree of contracture). If the hand can be placed flat on a surface (table top test) joint contracture will be minimal and operative treatment deferred. It is advisable to perform an Allen's test on digits that have been the site of previous surgery as vascular damage may have occurred. Knuckle pads known as Garrods nodes[8] over the dorsal aspect of the PIP joints are frequently encountered. The extent to which the skin is involved should be considered. Where there is widespread disease in a young patient with extensive skin tethering and dimpling a dermo-fasciectomy may be an appropriate procedure.

Radial club hand

History

The deformity may be mild or severe depending upon the state of the radius which can range from mild hypoplasia to complete absence. The condition usually arises sporadically but may be associated with a number of syndromes for example TAR syndrome (thrombocytopenia with absent radii which

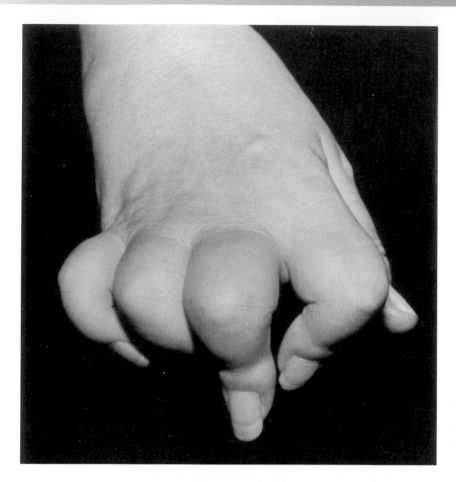

Figure 17 Psoriatic arthropathy with hyperextension deformities fo the MCP joints and fixed flexion deformities of the PIP joints.

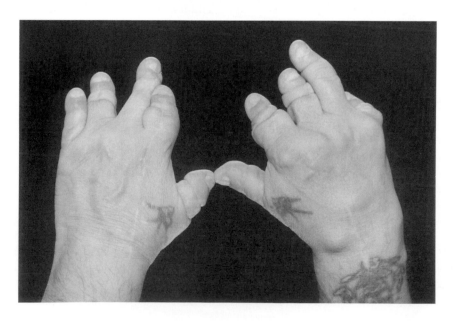

Figure 18 Collapsed skeleton of arthritis mutilans.

is always bilateral), Fanconi Anaemia (aplastic anaemia) and Holt-Oram syndrome (heart anomalies). Many occult abnormalities have been described which tend to come to light after careful screening. Occasionally a diagnosis is made on the antenatal ultrasound.

Examination

It is important to assess the movement of the shoulder and the elbow as these may affect the ability of the patient to put the hand to the mouth. The affected limb will be short and the ulnar in severe cases will be curved. Often the thumb is absent and the little finger is the most normal digit. Frequently the digits on the radial side of the hand are hypoplastic and stiff.

Assessment of the passive range of movement of the hand on the ulnar is important, as pre-surgical treatment will involve stretching of the tight radial structures using a small external fixator (**Figure 19**).

Syndactyly

History

Separate fingers are formed as a result of programmed cell death between the digits before the 8th week of gestation. Failure of this mechanism results in joined fingers. A positive family history is common and the condition is frequently bilateral. It may present as part of a syndrome e.g. Poland's or Apert's.

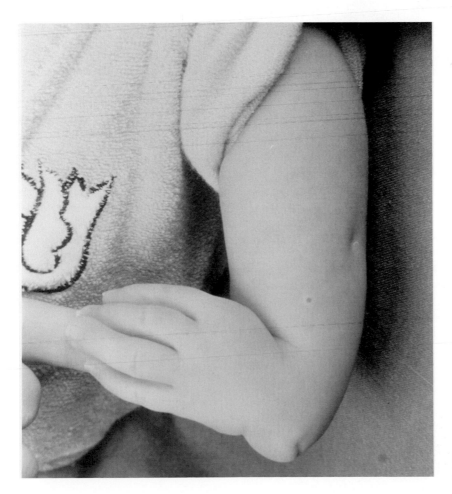

Figure 19 Radial club hand with absent thumb.

Examination

The condition is classified according to the position of the web as complete or incomplete. Then complex if the skeleton is in any way abnormal or simple if normal. The third web space is the most commonly involved. In complex cases the nail bed may be fused (**Figure 20**).

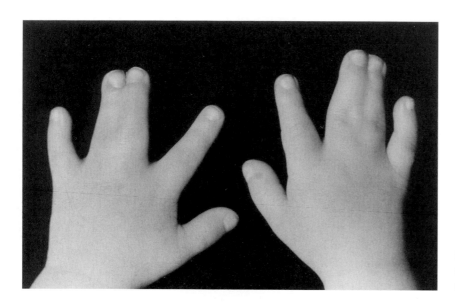

Figure 20 Bilateral complete simple syndactyly of both 3rd web spaces.

References

1. Reading G. Secretan's syndrome: hand oedema of the dorsum of the hand *Plast Reconstr Surg* 1980; **65:** 182–187

2. Leddy JP, Packer MD. Avulsion of the profundus tendon insertion in athletes *J Hand Surg 1977*; **2:** 66–69

3. Mannerfelt L, Norman O. Attrition ruptures of flexor tendons in rheumatoid arthritis caused by bony spurs in the carpal tunnel. *J Bone Joint Surg* 1969; **51:** 270–277

4. Vaughan-Jackson OJ. Rupture of extensor tendons by attrition at the inferior radio-ulnar joint. *J Bone Joint Surg* 1948; **30:** 528–530

5. Nalebuff EA, Millender LH. Surgical treatment of the swan-neck deformity in rheumatoid arthritis. *Orthop Clin North Am* 1975; **6:** 733–752

6. Nalebuff EA, Millender LH. Surgical treatment of the boutonniere deformity in rheumatoid arthritis. *Orthop Clin North Am* 1975; **6:** 753–763

7. Nalebuff EA. Diagnosis classification and management of rheumatoid thumb deformities. *Bull Hosp Jt Dis 1968*; **29:** 119–137

8. Garrod AE. Concerning pads upon the finger joints and their clinical relationships. *BMJ* 1875; **1:** 665

Examination of the Wrist

S H Bostock

History

Patients with wrist problems often have a paucity of clinical signs. Specific provocative tests can be both difficult to perform and equivocal in their interpretation. A thorough history is therefore essential.

The history should start by recording the age, occupation and handedness of the patient together with any affected recreational activities including sports and hobbies.

History of presenting complaint

The basic complaint needs to be established. Is it pain, weakness, a swelling, stiffness or a combination of these? Are there other symptoms? How long has there been a problem. Was there an injury or has the onset been insidious? What was the nature of the injury, was it a single event and if so did it receive treatment at the time?

The site and nature of *pain* should be established (**Figure 1**). The patient should be asked to try to localise it as accurately as possible (for example, by pointing). What is its nature; is it constant or intermittent, sharp, dull or "burning"? Is it worse with use and eased by rest? Are there particular movements that aggravate the pain such as turning taps, opening jars?

Stiffness may be a part of the presenting problem. If so, which movements are resrtricted? Is there associated discomfort and how does this interfere with the use of the arm in functional terms?

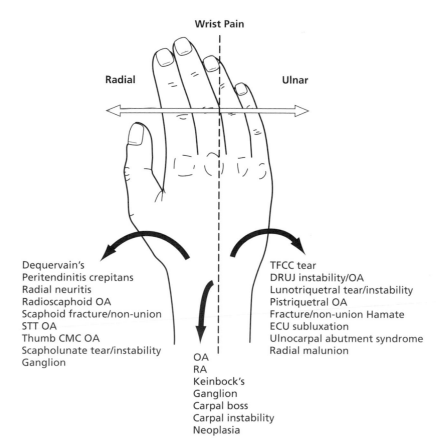

Wrist Pain

Radial   Ulnar

Dequervain's
Peritendinitis crepitans
Radial neuritis
Radioscaphoid OA
Scaphoid fracture/non-union
STT OA
Thumb CMC OA
Scapholunate tear/instability
Ganglion

OA
RA
Keinbock's
Ganglion
Carpal boss
Carpal instability
Neoplasia

TFCC tear
DRUJ instability/OA
Lunotriquetral tear/instability
Pistriquetral OA
Fracture/non-union Hamate
ECU subluxation
Ulnocarpal abutment syndrome
Radial malunion

Figure 1 Line drawing illustrating sites of commonly occurring pathologies about the wrist.

Swelling may be present. Is this the main problem? Is it painless ? Is the swelling growing or does its size vary?

Other symptoms may also be present; for example, a "click"or a "clunk". If so, is it painful? Has there been an injury? Is the wrist *weak*? Does the weakness appear to be secondary to pain?

The history also needs to document the impact that the patient's wrist problem has had on activities of daily living, work, sports and other hobbies.

Past medical history

It is important not to overlook the patient's past medical history. Have they had previous problems with this or the other wrist. If so, have they had surgery. Is there a history of arthritis. Is there a relevant family history?

Examination

Examination of the wrist should follow six basic steps:

1. Inspection
2. Palpation
3. Range of Motion
4. Provocative tests
5. General overview of the upper limb
6. Measurement of grip strength

1. Inspection

The patient should be sat comfortably in a chair directly facing the examiner. Patients will usually offer their wrist forward in pronation. Observe this and then place the opposite side in a corresponding position with the elbows to the sides. Look carefully and systematically at the wrists. Look at the overall alignment and shape of the forearm wrist and hand. Is there obvious deformity? What is the likely nature of this deformity (e.g. Madelung's deformity, Rheumatoid arthritis, Radial malunion)?

Rheumatoid arthritis[1]

Features:

- Extensor synovitis
- Extensor tendon rupture
- Dorsal subluxtion of the DRUJ
- Volar subluxation and supination of the carpus
- Ulnar translocation of the carpus with radial metacarpal drift and ulnar drift of the fingers
- Flexor synovitis
- Flexor tendon rupture
- Finger deformities
- Bilaterality
- Other joint involvement.

Radial malunion

Deformity most commonly follows the pattern of the original fracture. For example, radial shortening and prominence of the distal ulna.

Madelung's Deformity

Arises in childhood. Volar bowing of the distal radius, with dorsal prominence of the distal ulna. Look for hypoplastic radius, family history, absence of trauma, bilaterality. (Dorsal bowing may occur and is described as "Reverse Madelung's Deformity")

Now examine the wrist area in more detail. Starting on the dorsal aspect and working across from radial to ulnar. Is there fullness in the anatomical snuffbox? (Scaphoid pathology). Does the area around the radial styloid and first extensor compartment look swollen? (De Quervain's disease). Is there a swelling on the dorsum and if so what structure might this be overlying?

Dorsal wrist ganglion

Usually arise from and overlie the Scapholunate ligament[2] (just distal to Lister's tubercle).Will transilluminate if large. Pain without swelling in this area may represent an "Occult" ganglion.[3]

Carpal boss[4,5]

Bony hard swelling at the level of the 2nd and 3rd CMC joints dorsally. More distal than most simple ganglia. To confuse matters there may be an associated small overlying ganglion.

Extensor digitorum brevis manus

Extra (vestigial) muscle whose presence distal to the Extensor Retinaculum may confuse it with a ganglion or extensor synovitis. Moves with finger extension.

Are there any scars from previous surgery? If so what might have been done? What about the prominence of the distal ulna? Compare the two sides.

Once the dorsum has been inspected ask the patient to supinate. Is this movement painfree or restricted?

Carefully inspect this side of the wrist from its ulnar aspect back to radial, thus completing the circumference. Look for scars and swelling, comparing right with left.

Finally, fully flex the elbows and inspect the ulnar aspect of the wrists looking at the profile of the

Palpation

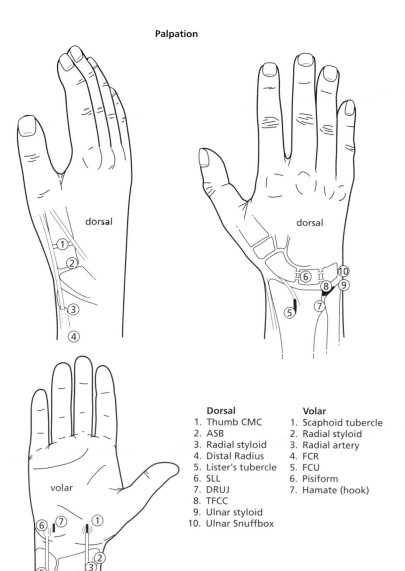

Dorsal	Volar
1. Thumb CMC	1. Scaphoid tubercle
2. ASB	2. Radial styloid
3. Radial styloid	3. Radial artery
4. Distal Radius	4. FCR
5. Lister's tubercle	5. FCU
6. SLL	6. Pisiform
7. DRUJ	7. Hamate (hook)
8. TFCC	
9. Ulnar styloid	
10. Ulnar Snuffbox	

Figure 2 Line drawing demonstrating a systematic approach to palpation around the wrist.

distal ulna in relation to the radius. Asymmetry suggests possible DRUJ subluxation (dorsal or volar).

2. Palpation

Palpation should also follow a system. Working across the wrist initially on it's dorsal aspect and then volarly (**Figure 2**). Palpation should be aimed at specific anatomic landmarks.

An attempt should be made to localise the area of tenderness as accurately as possible (**Figure 3**).

De Quervain's Disease

Swelling and pain localised to the first extensor compartment (Radial styloid). Crepitus may be present ("Wet leather sign"[6]). There may be an associated ganglion.

Radial Neuritis (Wartenberg's Neuralgia)

Pain and tenderness over the terminal cutaneous branches of the radial nerve. Look for a history of trauma.

Peritendinitis Crepitans (Intersection Syndrome)

Bursitis between APL/EPB and the wrist extensors (ECRL and ECRB). Crepitus is often palpable together with tenderness. This area of discomfort is more proximal than that in De Quervain's disease.

3. Range of Motion

Flexion / extension

This can be assessed by placing the palms of the hands together and lifting up the elbows (This allows for direct comparison of the right and left sides). Flexion can be measured in a similar way with the dorsum of both hands in apposition (**Figure 4**). A goniometer may be used to more accurately quantify the range. Each wrist is measured in turn. For wrist extension the goniometer is placed on the volar aspect in line with the radius and third metacarpal. For flexion, the goniometer is placed dorsally in the same line.

Radial and ulnar

Radial and ulnar deviation are assessed with the wrists in pronation and the elbows to the sides (**Figure 5**). The range can also be assessed with a

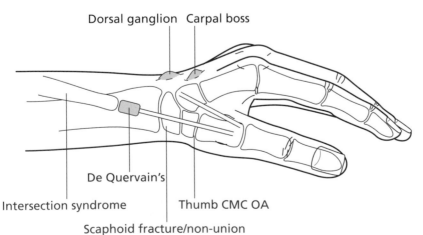

Dorsal ganglion   Carpal boss

De Quervain's

Intersection syndrome   Thumb CMC OA

Scaphoid fracture/non-union

Figure 3 Line drawing showing possible pathologies detectable by palpation over the radial aspect of the wrist.

Extension

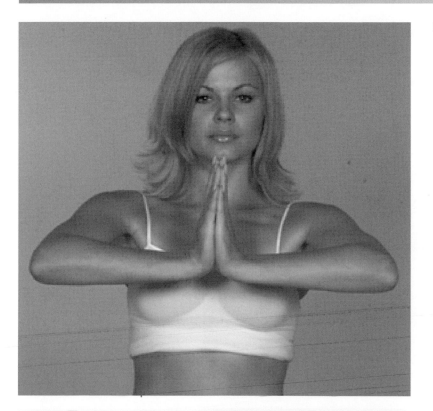

Flexion

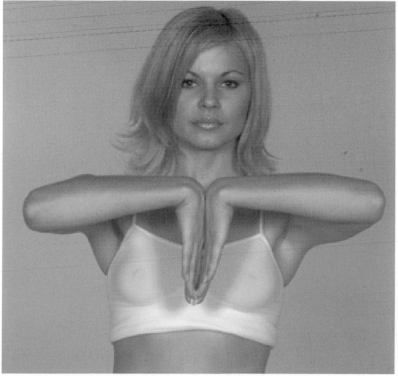

Figures 4 a,b Photographs showing simple way of assessing wrist extension and flexion.

Radial

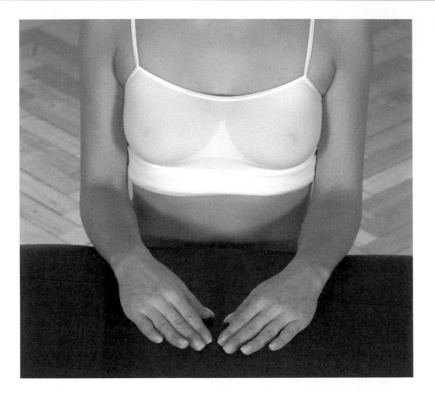

Ulnar

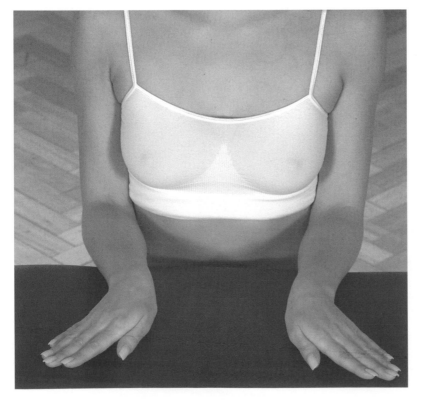

Figure 5 Photographs demonstrating radial and ulnar deviation.

goniometer by alignment with the radius and the third metacarpal on the dorsum of the wrist.

Pronation and supination

This is assessed with the elbows to the sides (**Figure 6**), again with a comparison of sides.

On occasions it may be appropriate to assess "active" range of motion in addition to the passive measurements.

4. Provocative Tests

A number of provocative tests for various conditions about the wrist have been described (**Table 1**). Clearly it would be inappropriate to perform all the available tests in every patient. Some sort of strategy is needed based on the history and examination thus far.

Finklestein's test[7]

The examiner supports the forearm with one hand. With the other hand the thumb is adducted and the wrist ulnarly deviated to put tension on the APL and EPB tendons (**Figure 7**). A positive test will elicit pain over the inflamed area in the region of the radial styloid

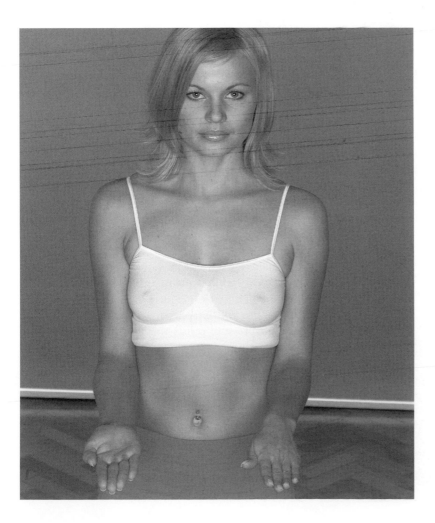

Figure 6 Photograph demonstrating pronation (left hand) and supination (right hand).

Table 1 Provocative Tests

Condition	Test
DeQuervain's	Finklestein's
Scapho-lunate instability	Scaphoid shift (Kirk Watson)
	Scaphoid thrust
	Scaphoid lift
Midcarpal instability	Midcarpal shift
	Pivot shift
Luno-triquetral instability	Ballotment (Reagan)
	Shear
	Compression
Ulnar sided pathology	Ulnocarpal stress
Pisotriquetral arthritis	Grind
DRUJ instability	Piano key
	Radio-ulnar drawer test
	Compression
	Dimple sign
ECU subluxation	
Hamate fracture/ non-union	

Carpal instability

A term which is used to describe a wide variety of pathological conditions, all of which stem from disruption of the complex ligament system that controls the relative motion of the bones that form the Carpus. A considerable number of instability patterns have been described. Provocative tests exist for Scapholunate, Lunotriquetral and Midcarpal Instability.

Scapholunate instability

Rupture of the scapho-lunate ligament permits abnormal movement between the Scaphoid and the Lunate. Kirk Watson described a provocative test to reproduce and clinically detect this abnormal movement. This test is known variously as the "Kirk Watson test", the "Watson test", the "Scaphoid test" or the "Scaphoid Shift".[8] Two other tests for Scapholunate instability are the "Scaphoid Thrust" and the "Scaphoid Lift" tests.[9,10]

Scaphoid shift test (Kirk Watson)[8]

The examiner uses one hand to grasp the wrist, placing the fingers dorsally (index or middle finger tips to lie over the area of the scapholunate ligament). The thumb is placed over the scaphoid tubercle volarly. With the examiner's other hand the patient's wrist is moved from radial into ulnar deviation whilst maintaining pressure on the scaphoid tubercle (**Figures 8** and **9**). With radial deviation the scaphoid will usually flex. The thumb pressure resists this and in the presence of a scapholunate tear the scaphoid subluxes dorsally off the radius. A positive test occurs when this abnormal movement is felt by the examiner, often as a "click". Pain may also be a significant finding, but is less specific for scapholunate instability. The Scaphoid Shift is positive in up to 36% of "normal" individuals.[11]

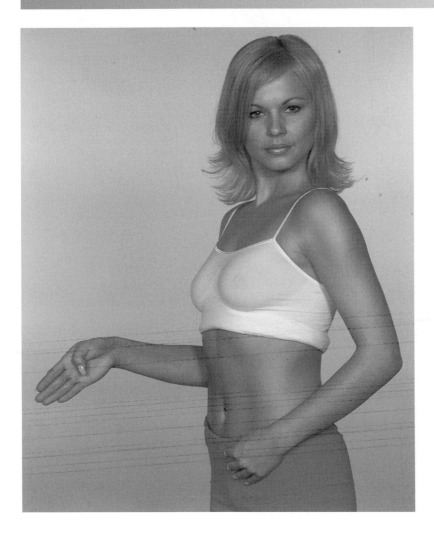

Figure 7 Photograph demonstrating Finklestein's Test which stresses the first extensor compartment, a provocative test for De Quervain's tenosynovitis.

Scaphoid thrust test[9]

Lane has described a modification of the Kirk Watson test which he originally, rather confusingly, named the scaphoid shift test, but which has been renamed the scaphoid Thrust test. The patient's hand is held in the same way as for the scaphoid shift with the examiner's thumb over the scaphoid tubercle. The wrist is rocked backwards and forwards from radial to ulnar deviation and back again until the patient is relaxed and guarding has been eliminated. The sacphoid tubercle is then quickly pressed by the examiners thumb with the wrist in slight radial deviation and neutral flexion/extension. For a positive test the scaphoid should be felt to move dorsally.

Scaphoid lift test[10]

A third test has been described in which the Lunate is stabilised with the thumb and index finger of one hand whilst the scaphoid is translocated volarly and dorsally using the other thumb and index finger.

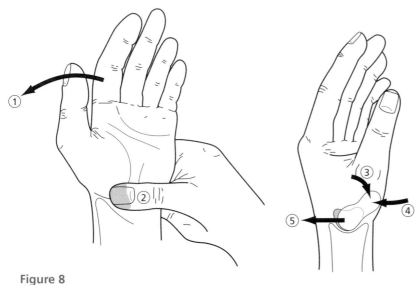

1. The wrist is moved from ulnar into radial deviation
2. Pressure is applied by the examiner's thumb to resist Scaphoid flexion
3. Scaphoid rotates (flexes) with radial deviation of the wrist
4. Applied force (examiner's thumb)
5. Subluxation (may be felt by examiner's index/middle finger)

Figure 8

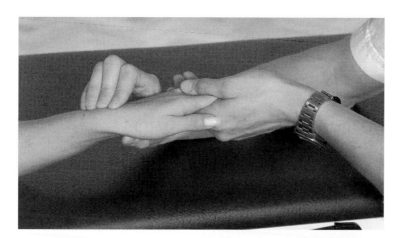

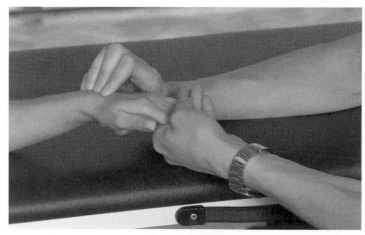

Figure 9

Figures 8 & 9 These illustrations demonstrate the scaphoid shift test. Pressure over the scaphoid tubercle with the examiner's thumb whilst radially deviating the wrist causes a click or pain in scapholunate instability.

Midcarpal instability

The "Drawer tests" may be positive in patients with midcarpal instability, although are more commonly an assessment of general ligamentous laxity. More specific tests for midcarpal instability are the "Midcarpal Shift test" and the "Pivot Shift"

Radiocarpal and midcarpal drawer tests

The examiner firmly grasps the patient's forearm with one hand. With the other hand the patient's hand is held at metacarpal level and a distracting force is applied. A dorsal and volar translating force is then applied and the amount of movement assessed (comparing sides). If the examiner then repeats the manoeuvre but moves his distal hand proximally to the level of the proximal carpal row it has been suggested that it is possible to assess laxity across the midcarpal joint.

Midcarpal shift test[10,12]

The examiner stabilises the forearm with one hand. With his other hand the examiner places his thumb over the capitate dorsally. A volarly directed force is applied as the wrist is ulnarly deviated. If there is a palpable "clunk" as the wrist approaches full ulnar deviation then this is a positive test. The degree of laxity and clunking has been graded (I-V). It is thought that in patient's with midcarpal instability the proximal carpal row is slow to dorsiflex as the wrist ulnarly deviates and that the clunk represents a catch up movement.

A slight variation on this test applies an axial rather than a volar load as the wrist is ulnarly deviated.

Pivot shift test[13, 14]

The elbow is placed on a firm surface and the hand is fully supinated. The forearm is held firmly. The hand is radially deviated and pressure applied to the dorso-ulnar aspect of the carpus. The hand is then ulnarly deviated . A normal wrist "Notches" into a less supinated position as the capitate engages the lunate.

Ulnar sided wrist pain

The diagnosis of ulnar sided wrist pain is difficult. The Ulnocarpal stress test[15] is a general screening test for ulnar sided pathology. More specific tests have been described to try and separate out the underlying pathology.

Difficulty arises not least because of the interrelationship between the different processes. For example, ulnocarpal impingement may be associated with a TFCC tear. The TFCC is a stabiliser of the DRUJ and a tear may therefore be associated with painful instability of the DRUJ. Thus in the context of clinical examination it may be impossible and inaccurate to try to establish a single diagnosis.

Ulnocarpal stress test[15]

With the forearm supported the examiner applies axial load to the wrist, which is held in ulnar deviation and neutral flexion/extension. The forearm is then rotated (**Figure 10**). A positive test elicits pain on the ulnar side of the wrist.

A variation of this test is to hold the forearm with the wrist in neutral pronation and supination but ulnar deviation. The wrist is then flexed and extended. A positive test elicits pain.

Lunotriquetral ligament injuries (instability)

Carpal instability associated with predominantly ulnar sided symptoms may be secondary to a lunotriquetral ligament tear. Reagan et al. have described a Ballotment Test[16]. There are also Compression and Shear tests whilst three other tests have been described by Christodoulou and Bainbridge[17].

Ballotment test (Reagan)[16]

The lunate is fixed between the thumb and index finger of one hand. With the other thumb and index finger the triqetrum (and pisiform) are displaced dorsally and volarly (**Figure 11**). Laxity, pain or crepitus indicates a positive result.

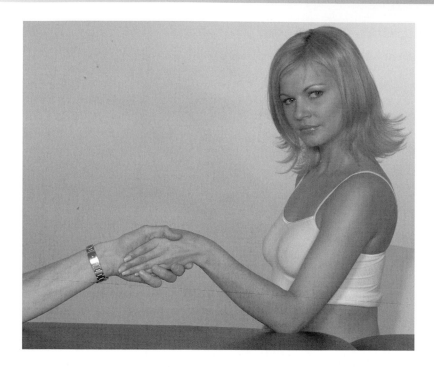

Figure 10 Photograph showing Ulnocarpal Stress Test. This is a general screening test for ulnar sided pathology.

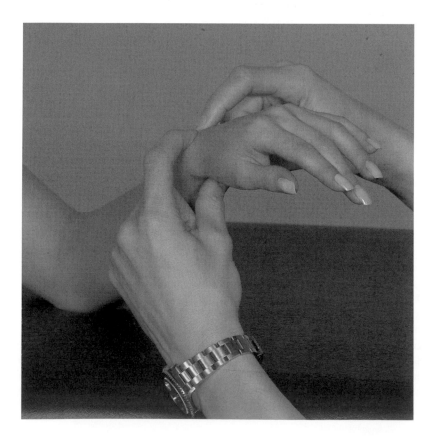

Figure 11 Photograph demonstrating Ballotment Test. Fixing the lunate between the finger and thumb of one hand and displacing the triquetrum dorsally and volarly with the other causes pain or demonstrates laxity in patients with lunotriquetral instability.

Shear test

The Lunate is stabilised with the thumb over the dorsal aspect of the wrist. A force is the applied to the Pisiform volarly, thus indirectly applying a shear force across the Lunotriquetral joint.

Compression

Pressure is applied over the "ulnar snuffbox" (between ECU and FCU and distal to the ulna styloid). This loads the triquetrolunate (and Triquetrohamate) joints.

Other Tests

Chistodoulou and Bainbridge[17]describe three further tests. In the first of these the wrist is dorsiflexed, radially deviated and the forearm fully pronated. The examiner's thumb pushes against the pisiform whilst the fingers apply counter-pressure over the distal ulna. Whilst this pressure is maintained the wrist is brought into a neutral position. A positive result elicits pain and sometimes a click as the pisiform "reduces"during this manoeuvre.

Pisotriquetral arthritis

Pisotriquetral arthritis is a cause of ulnar sided wrist pain. Many of the tests described for lunotriquetral tears apply compression across the pisotriquetral joint and these tests are likely to be positive for pain where there is arthritis. A Grind test has also been described.

Grind test

In this the pisiform is held between the thumb and index finger. Compression is applied and the pisiform displaced back and forth in a radial and ulnar direction.

The distal radioulnar joint:

Problems with the distal radioulnar joint may be isolated or part of a complex of injuries. Pain on pronation and supination may be exacerbated by Compression. The (Radioulnar) Drawer test, "Piano Key" test and "Dimple Sign" may indicate joint subluxation.

Compression test

Pain on pronation and supination of the forearm may not be specific to the distal radioulnar joint. The compression test applies a force across the joint by squeezing the forearm which is then pronated and supinated. A positive test occurs where this increases pain in the region of the DRUJ.

Piano key test (Figure 12)

The examiner stabilises the forearm distally with his fingers over the volar aspect. The thumb then presses over the distal ulna. Increased excursion suggests dorsal subluxation (e.g. RA)

Radioulnar drawer test

The flexed elbow is rested on a firm surface. The radius is stabilised with one hand. The ulna is grasped between the fingers and thumb of the other hand and moved dorsally and volarly. This can be repeated with the forearm in different positions of pronation and supination and should be compared with the opposite side. Laxity of the DRUJ can be assessed and if excessive may be a sign of instability, especially if this is associated with discomfort.

Dimple sign

Longitudinal traction is applied across the wrist. A force is applied to the dorsal aspect of the ulna shaft. If a "dimple" appears at the level of the DRUJ then this suggests volar subluxation.

ECU subluxation

Subluxation of the ECU tendon may be provoked by placing the forearm in supination and ulnar deviation. With dorsiflexion the tendon may be painful and can sometimes be felt to sublux volarly.

Hamate fracture / Non–union

Tenderness over the hook of the Hamate (distal and radial to the Pisiform) may indicate an underlying fracture or non-union. In these condi-

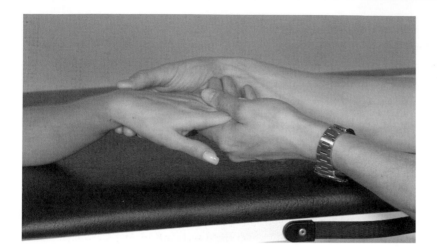

Figure 12 This photograph demonstrates the piano key test. Pressure over the ulnar styloid by the examiner's thumb in a dorsal to volar direction will demonstrate increased excursion in patients with dorsal subluxation.

tions the pain may be made worse by resisted flexion of the little and ring fingers with the wrist in ulnar deviation.

5. Overview of the Upper Limb

The wrist should not be considered in isolation. Some attention needs to be paid to the upper limb in general.

The neurological status:	Briefly assess motor and sensory function.
Vascular status:	Palpate radial artery. Allen's test.
Other Joints:	Briefly assess the shoulder, elbow and hand.

6. Measurement of Grip Strength

Grip strength can be measured using a Jamar dynamometer. This provides an objective measurement of one aspect of hand function.

With the shoulder adducted and the elbow flexed to 90 degrees the patient is asked to squeeze the dynamometer with maximum strength. The test is repeated three times for each wrist. A "rapid exchange" technique has been described to detect submaximal effort.[18]

References

1. Taleisnik J. *The Wrist*. Churchill Livingstone 1986.

2. Angelides AC, Wallace PF. The dorsal ganglion of the wrist: Its pathogenesis, gross and microscopic anatomy, and surgical treatment. *J Hand Surg [Am]* 1976; **1(3):** 228–235.

3. Sanders WE. The occult dorsal carpal ganglion. *J Hand Surg [B]* 1985; **10-B(2):** 257–260.

4. Clarke AM, Wheen DJ, Visvanathan S, Herbert TJ, Conolly WB. The symptomatic carpal boss. Is simple excision enough. *J Hand Surg [B] 1999;* **24-B(5):** 591–595.

5. Cuono CB, Watson HK. The carpal boss: Surgical treatment and aetiological considerations. *Plas Reconstr Surg 1979;* **63:** 88–93.

6. Green DP, Hotchkiss MD, Pederson WC. *Green's Operative Hand Surgery* (4th ed.). Churchill Livingstone 1998.

7. Finklestein H. Stenosing tendovaginitis of the radial styloid process. *J Bone Joint Surg [Am]* 1930; **12-A:** 509–540.

8. Watson HK, Ashmead D, Makhlouf MV. Examination of the scaphoid. *J Hand Surg [A]* 1988; **13-A(5):** 657–660.

9. Lane LB. The scaphoid shift test. *J Hand Surg [A]* 1993; **18(A):** 366–368.

10. Cooney WP, Linscheid RL, Dobyns J. *The Wrist: Diagnosis and Operative Treatment*. Mosby 1998.

11. Easterling KJ, Wolfe SW. Scaphoid shift in the uninjured wrist. *J Hand Surg [A]* 1994; **19-A(4):** 604–606.

12. Feinstein WK, Lichtman DM, Noble PC, Alexander JW, Hipp JA. Quantitative assessment of the midcarpal shift test. *J Hand Surg [A]* 1999; **24-A (5):** 977– 983.

13. Tubiana R, Thomine J, Mackin E. *Examination of the Hand and Wrist*. Martin Dunitz 1998.

14. Stanley J, Saffar P. *Wrist Arthroscopy*. Martin Dunitz 1994.

15. Nakamura R, Horii E, Imaeda T, Nakao E, Kato H, Watanabe K. The ulnocarpal stress test in the diagnosis of ulnar-sided wrist pain. *J Hand Surg [B]* 1997; **22-B (6):** 719–723.

16. Reagan DS, Linscheid RL, Dobyns JH. Lunotriquetral sprains. *J Hand Surg [A]* 1984; **9-A(4):** 502–514.

17. Christodoulou L, Bainbridge LC. Clinical diagnosis of Triquetrolunate ligament injuries. *J hand Surg [B]* 1999; **24-B (5):** 598–600.

18. Hildreth DH, Breidenbach WC, Lister GD, Hodges AD. Detection of submaximal effort by use of the rapid exchange grip. *J Hand Surg [A]* 1989; **14-A:** 742–745.

3

Clinical Examination of the Elbow

D Stanley

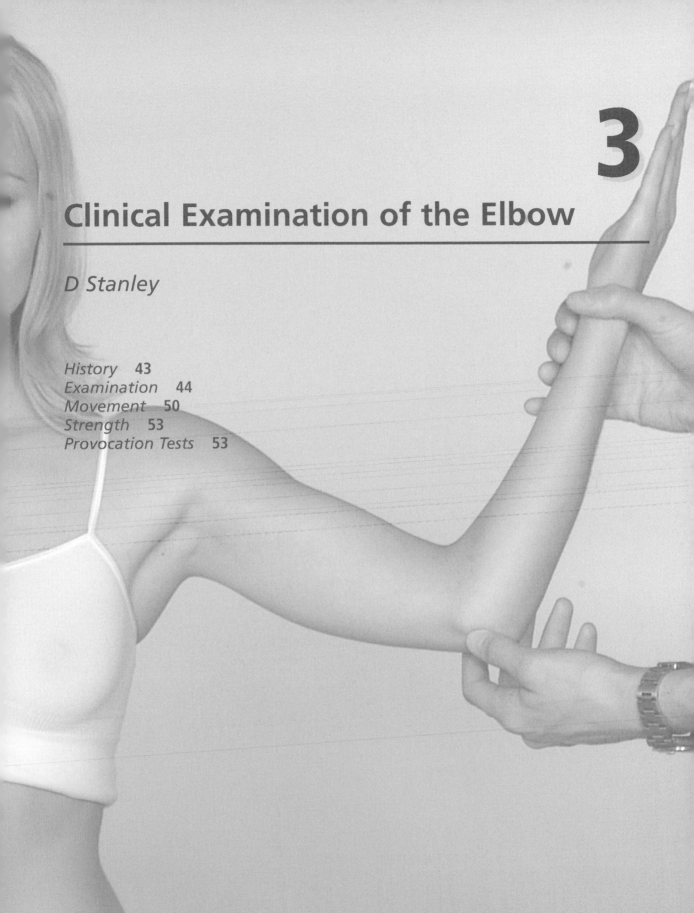

As with the examination of all other joints in the body a carefully taken and detailed clinical history will often lead the clinician to a provisional diagnosis of the cause of the patient's elbow problem.

As the patient describes the symptoms the clinician should be interpreting the information in the light of the local anatomy, most of which, because the elbow is a superficial joint, can be palpated and assessed during the examination.

History

It is always essential when taking a history to record the patient's age, sex and hand dominance.

Age will give an immediate clue as to the likelihood of certain conditions being responsible for the patient's complaints. For example osteochondritis dissecans may be the underlying cause of elbow locking in a young patient whereas the same symptoms in an older patient are more likely to be due to loose body formation associated with degenerative disease.

The elbow may be the first presenting site of rheumatoid arthritis, and since this occurs more commonly in women the sex of the patient should alert one to the possibility of this diagnosis if the initial symptoms are pain and slight swelling.

Hand dominance is of importance since a disorder of the dominant elbow may result in the patient's inability to work, participate in sporting activity or undertake activities of daily living.

In addition to the current symptoms it is important to enquire about the patient's previous medical health particularly with regards to whether there is any history of previous similar problems. Enquiry should also be made with regards previous trauma, occupation and current sporting activity.[1]

Presenting symptoms

Most patients with elbow disorders present with pain, often associated with tenderness, or reduced elbow movement. In addition intermittent swelling and locking may also occur. More unusually recurrent instability of the elbow is a significant problem. Combinations of these symptoms are not infrequent.

The nature of the patient's pain together with its location and frequency should be noted. It is important to record whether the pain is associated with movement and whether or not there is a history of pain radiation. For example patients with ulnar nerve entrapment may experience local pain and tenderness at the elbow together with pain radiation down into the hand affecting the little and ring fingers, often with intermittent pins and needles or numbness.

Reduced elbow movement can be the result of a variety of conditions but perhaps more commonly is seen after elbow trauma or as a result of degenerative and inflammatory arthropathies. Loose bodies within the elbow joint may be another cause of reduced elbow movement and this pathology is also often associated with intermittent elbow locking.

Although rare recurrent instability of the elbow does occur following elbow trauma particularly if the coronoid process has been damaged or the collateral ligaments torn. Instability may also be a feature of inflammatory arthropathy especially when the disease has resulted in significant bony destruction.

Symptoms of crepitus are not often reported by the patient and should be specifically asked about since this may indicate mechanical derangement of the elbow or an inflammatory arthropathy.

As with all upper limb disorders it is essential to specifically ask the patient about neck symptoms since at times cervical spine pathology may result in symptoms referable to the elbow.

Previous medical history

A review of the patient's past medical history should enquire specifically about previous similar symptoms and previous elbow trauma. It is also important to ask about other joint injuries which may have an effect on the elbow and to enquire about symptoms suggestive of chronic inflammatory disease.

At times elbow pain may be a feature of a generalised 'mesenchymal syndrome'. This occurs particularly in women in the fourth decade of life. The elbow symptoms include lateral and medial epicondylitis and may also involve ulnar nerve compression at the elbow. The symptoms are, however, not limited to the elbow region and such patients will frequently have shoulder symptoms together with wrist and hand problems such as carpal tunnel syndrome and stenosing tenovaginitis of the fingers and thumbs.

General health

It is of relevance to enquire about the patient's general health since this may indicate a generalised musculo-skeletal disorder. In addition, enquiry as to the patient's family history may reveal problems such as haemophilia or osteochondromatosis.

The patient's occupation is of relevance since there is some evidence to suggest that heavy manual work may be associated with degenerative change within the elbow joint.[2] Similarly an enquiry with regards sporting activity is of importance. Throwing athletes may develop symptoms of ulnar collateral ligament insufficiency occurring primarily during the late cocking and early acceleration phases of the throwing movement. Other athletes who undertake recurrent flexion and extension movements of the elbow i.e. boxers may develop posterior elbow impingement due to recurrent impact of the tip of the olecranon into the olecranon fossa.

Examination

Inspection

It is important to note the posture in which the patient holds the elbow. A painful elbow will often be protected with the arm being held adjacent to the patient's body whilst patients who are unable to fully extend the elbow often find it most comfortable resting the arm by placing the hand in a trouser pocket.

Inspection should also include a close assessment of the elbow for evidence of previous scars either traumatic or surgical or the presence of elbow swelling such as will occur with an acute injury, inflammatory arthritis or a neoplastic lesion. Rheumatoid nodules may be noted on the extensor aspect of the elbow.

Palpation

A systematic approach to examination of the elbow must be developed. Much of the elbow is subcutaneous and therefore by careful examination most of the structures likely to be causing the patient's symptoms can be individually examined and assessed.

The lateral and anterior aspects of the elbow can be palpated with the examiner standing in front of the patient whilst the medial and posterior aspects of the elbow are best examined from behind with the shoulder slightly abducted and extended.

Lateral

Examination of the lateral aspect of the elbow joint begins at the lateral supracondylar ridge (**Figure 1**). This is easily palpable. Examination should extend down the ridge to the lateral epicondyle, common extensor origin and lateral collateral ligament.

The extensor carpi radialis brevis and extensor carpi radialis longus muscles can be assessed by resisted wrist extension in neutral and radial deviation respectively. Tenderness particularly at the site of the extensor carpi radialis brevis should alert the clinician to a possible diagnosis of lateral epicondylitis.[3]

The capitellar joint line should be palpated since tenderness and discomfort at this site may indicate an articular injury or the presence of osteochondritis dissecans.

Inspection of the infra-condylar recess between the lateral condyle and radial head will normally reveal a small sulcus. This is obliterated by fluid or synovial distention. Palpation of the area will reveal a boggy swelling if due to synovial hypertrophy while fluctuation is noted if fluid is within the joint.

The radial head is best appreciated during pronation and supination movement of the forearm. The

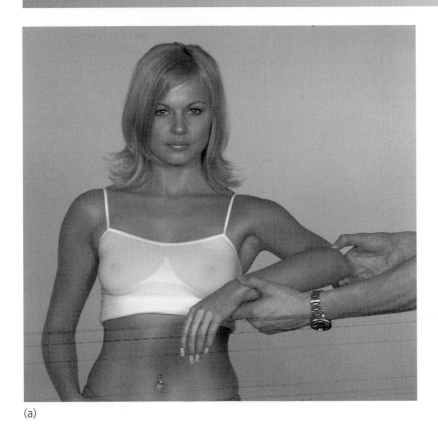

(a)

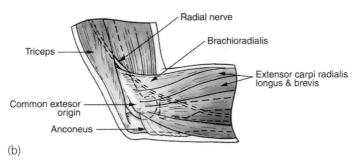

Triceps

Radial nerve

Brachioradialis

Extensor carpi radialis longus & brevis

Common extesor origin

Anconeus

(b)

Figure 1 (a) Examination of the lateral aspect of the elbow. (b) The anatomy of the lateral aspect of the elbow.

orientation of the radial head to the capitellum should be determined and in all positions of the elbow and forearm the radial head should line up against the capitellum. Congenital or post-traumatic dislocation of the radial head (lateral, posterior or anterior) will be easily appreciated at this stage.[4]

In the presence of a recent injury palpable crepitus over the radial head together with pain on rotation movements of the forearm is usually indicative of a radial head fracture although at times there may also be an associated capitellar injury. In the absence of a recent injury pain and crepitus at the radio-capitellar joint is usually indicative of degenerative change. The symptoms may be exacerbated by asking the patient to grip the examiner's fingers during forearm rotation.

Anterior

Anteriorly the brachio-radialis muscle, the biceps tendon together with the lacertus fibrosus, the brachial artery and the median nerve can be palpated from lateral to medial (**Figure 2**).

Although uncommon myositis ossificans may occur after elbow dislocation and may be palpated as an abnormal hard swelling during examination of the anterior aspect of the elbow joint.[5]

Another uncommon condition that may be appreciated on anterior elbow palpation is rupture of the insertion of the biceps tendon[6] (**Figure 3**). The patient will normally present with a history of recent injury and examination of the arm reveals a retracted biceps with the muscle bulge appearing more proximally in the arm as opposed to the more

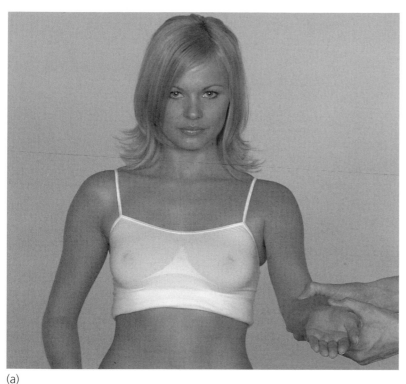

(a)

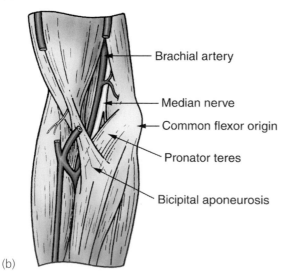

—— Brachial artery

—— Median nerve

—— Common flexor origin

—— Pronator teres

—— Bicipital aponeurosis

(b)

Figure 2 (a) Examination of the anterior aspect of the elbow. (b) The anatomy of the anterior aspect of the elbow.

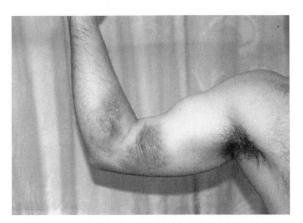

Figure 3 Rupture of the Insertion of the Biceps. Note the proximal position of the biceps muscle.

common long head of biceps rupture where the muscle bulge is distal. Assessment of flexor power and particularly supination power will indicate significant reduction when compared to the uninjured side.

Medial

Tenderness on palpation of the medial epicondyle and origin of the common flexors will indicate medial epicondylitis whilst tenderness over the belly of pronator teres should suggest the diagnosis of pronator syndrome.[7] Clinical features of this syndrome are often rather vague. They consist primarily of diffuse proximal forearm discomfort and weakness which, in addition, may be associated with distal sensory changes in the distribution of the median nerve. Phalen's test and Tinel's sign are negative at the wrist whilst percussion over the median nerve at the elbow results in tingling distally.

Provocation tests, when positive, are helpful in confirming the diagnosis. These include resisted pronation for 60 seconds, resisted elbow flexion and forearm supination and resisted middle finger flexion at the proximal interphalangeal joint.

The ulnar nerve should be palpated and can be easily felt behind the medial epicondyle (**Figure 4**). It should be remembered that in up to 10% of patients the ulnar nerve may sublux anteriorly and it is important to identify the position of the ulnar nerve during flexion and extension movements of the elbow. A subluxing ulnar nerve may give rise to medial elbow pain.

More commonly compression of the ulnar nerve gives rise to sensory and/or motor symptoms.[8]

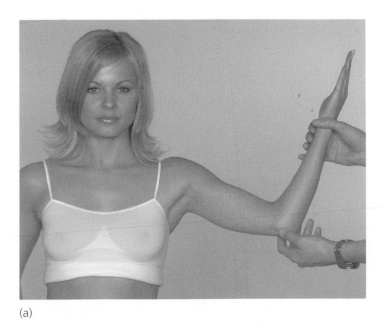

(a)

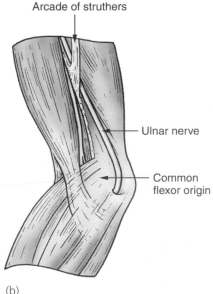

Arcade of struthers

Ulnar nerve

Common flexor origin

(b)

Figure 4 (a) Examination of the medial aspect of the elbow. (b) The anatomy of the medial aspect of the elbow.

These may occur secondary to degenerative or inflammatory arthritis, medial epicondylitis, elbow instability and fracture dislocations. The nerve is most commonly compressed at the cubital tunnel and between the two heads of flexor carpi ulnaris. Tinel's sign is usually positive at the point of maximal nerve tenderness.

Posterior

With the elbow extended the tip of the olecranon process and the medial and lateral epicondyles form a straight line. On flexion of the elbow to 90° these landmarks form an isosceles triangle (**Figure 5**). Any abnormality of this normal arrangement is suggestive of previous bony injury.

With the arm extended the triceps insertion onto the olecranon can be palpated and the integrity of the triceps tested by resisted extension (**Figure 6**). Tenderness on this manoeuvre may represent a partial tear of the triceps whilst an inability to extend against gravity is indicative of a complete triceps avulsion.[9]

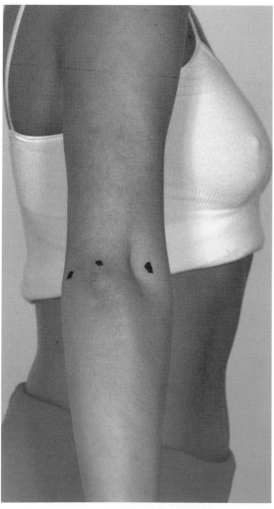

(a)

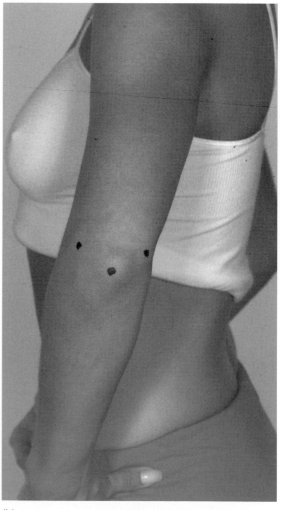

(b)

Figure 5 The bony relationship of the tip of the olecranon process to the medial and lateral epicondyles (a) With the elbow extended it is a horizontal line; and (b) With the elbow flexed to 90° an isosceles triangle is formed.

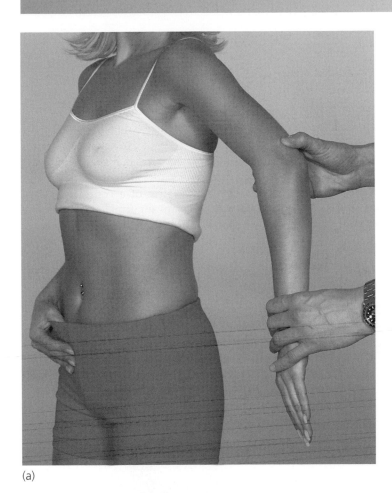

(a)

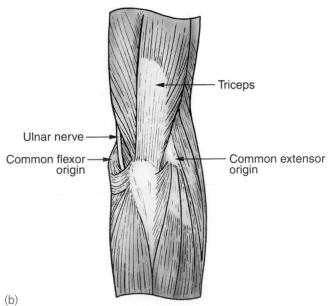

Triceps

Ulnar nerve

Common flexor origin

Common extensor origin

(b)

Figure 6 (a) Examination of the posterior aspect of the elbow. (b) The anatomy of the posterior aspect of the elbow.

The olecranon fossa can be palpated with the elbow flexed to 30°. In the thin patient it is occasionally possible to palpate a loose body within the fossa.

Examination of the olecranon bursa may reveal a bursitis or indicate the presence of rheumatoid nodules.

Movement

Movement of the elbow can only adequately be assessed in a patient whose top clothes have been removed. It is important to compare both upper limbs in order to clearly identify subtle changes in elbow movement.

Axial alignment

The elbow carrying angle should be assessed with the elbow in full extension. If this is not possible due to elbow pathology then the assessment of the carrying angle is compromised.

Although the carrying angle varies the average valgus angulation is 10° in males and 15° in females. An increase in valgus angulation may result from a previous bony injury to the lateral distal humerus.

Varus deformity is always abnormal and most commonly occurs as the result of a supracondylar fracture in childhood or a growth arrest on the medial side of the distal humerus.

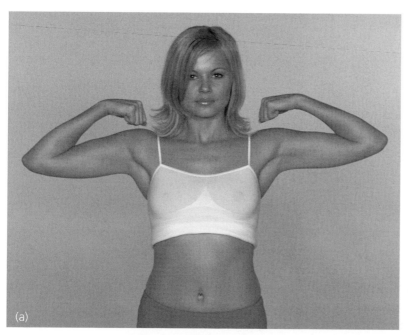

(a)

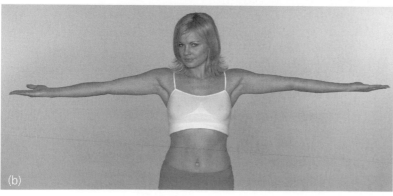

(b)

Figure 7 The range of flexion (a) and extension (b) in the normal elbow.

It should be noted that when the elbow is flexed from the fully extended position the carrying angle changes from being valgus to varus.[10]

Flexion / extension

With the forearms supinated and extended the normal range of movement is from 0–140° of flexion (**Figure 7**). Up to 10° of hyperextension (recorded as a negative integer) is not abnormal but hyperextension beyond that level is suggestive of hyper mobility or previous bony injury.

Loss of full extension is often the earliest sign of an intra-articular elbow abnormality.

A discrepancy between the passive and active range of movement is suggestive of either a musculo-tendinous or neurological abnormality.

Forearm rotation

Forearm rotation is assessed with both elbows flexed to 90° and with the arms adducted to the body (**Figure 8**). This prevents compensatory shoulder movement.

Variation in supination and pronation movement occurs in normal patients although the average range of supination is 85° whilst pronation is normally a few degrees less.

Rotational deformity

Rotational deformity is often not appreciated and results from either an abnormality of the shoulder or humerus.

If both shoulders are normal an asymmetric range

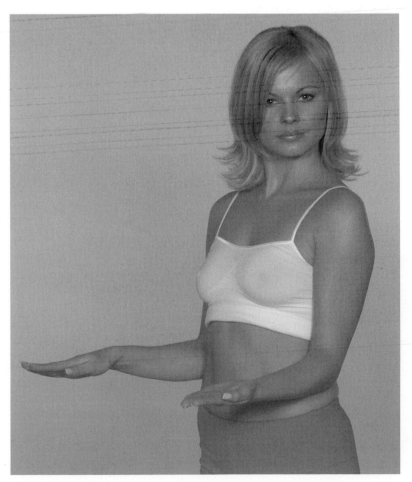

Figure 8 The range of pronation (right hand) and supination (left hand) in the normal elbow.

of rotation is indicative of a humeral rotational deformity. This may result from previous humeral fractures.

The deformity is best demonstrated by the technique described by Yamamoto et al[11] (**Figure 9**).

The examiner stands behind the patient with the elbow flexed to 90° and the forearm behind the back. With the patient bent forward and the shoulder in full extension the forearm is lifted maximally resulting in maximal internal rotation. Difference in the internal rotation angle of the two arms can be measured by the angle between the forearm and the horizontal of the back. This angle is frequently increased in mal-united supracondylar fractures.

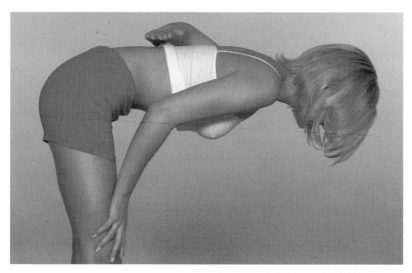

(a)

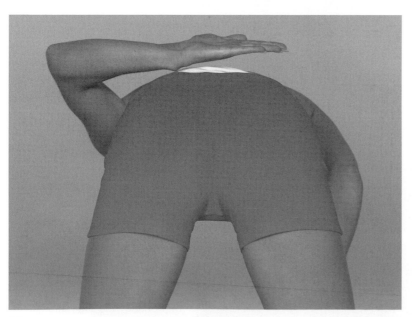

(b)

Figure 9 The assessment of rotational deformity. The patient is bent forward. The shoulder fully extended and the elbow flexed to 90°. If there is no rotational deformity the forearm is parallel to the ground (a). If there is Increased internal rotation in the humerus then the acute angle between the line of the forearm and the horizontal gives a measure of the internal rotation deformity (b).

Strength

Although detailed assessment of muscle strength is not possible in the setting of the consulting room it is possible to obtain a gross assessment of muscle strength by comparing both arms.

Flexion is tested with the elbow flexed to 90° and the forearm in neutral rotation. Resistance to the flexion movement is applied and the two arms compared.

Extension is tested with the arm in a similar position but on this occasion resistance to extension movement is provided.

Pronation and supination strength is assessed with the elbows flexed to 90° and in neutral rotation. The movement under test is resisted. Normally supination is slightly stronger than pronation.

Provocation Tests

Lateral epicondylitis

Specific provocation tests that can be performed in order to help confirm the diagnosis are as follows:[12]

1. With the wrist in neutral resisted wrist extension results in localised pain over the lateral epicondyle. Pain may also occur if the test is undertaken with the wrist in extension and radial deviation and on resisted extension of the middle finger (**Figure 10**).
2. Passive volar flexion of the wrist with elbow extension and pronation will also cause pain at the lateral epicondyle. Pinch grip particularly between the thumb and middle finger is often weak and painful.

If the patient's symptoms and signs suggest lateral epicondylitis and if the above provocative tests are positive then an injection of a small volume of local anaesthetic at the attachment of the extensor carpi radialis brevis will often confirm the diagnosis by eliminating the symptoms. Failure of improvement to occur should lead to re-assessment of the diagnosis.

It is important that care is taken during the performance of such an injection since if local anaesthetic goes into the elbow joint and obliterates the symptoms a wrong diagnosis will be made.

Medial epicondylitis

This is characterised by tenderness of the common flexor origin at the medial epicondyle. Provocation tests include:

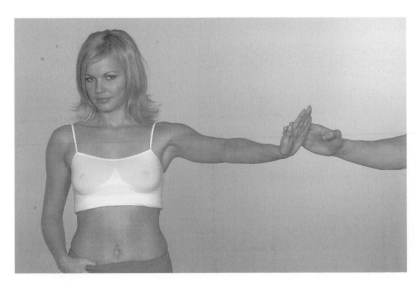

Figure 10 Provocation testing for lateral epicondylitis.

1. Resisted wrist flexion causes pain at the medial epicondyle (**Figure 11**).
2. Passive extension of the wrist and elbow results in pain at the medial epicondyle.
3. Clenching of the fist may also cause pain at the medial epicondyle.

In the same way that injection of local anaesthetic at the lateral epicondyle can be beneficial, injection of a small quantity of local anaesthetic at the site of maximal medial epicondyle pain should also obliterate the symptoms.

Impingement

Elbow impingement most commonly occurs in the posterior compartment of the elbow joint but can also occur anteriorly.

In the posterior compartment the symptoms are normally associated with osteophytic changes at the tip of the olecranon which impinge on the olecranon fossa during extension. Loose bodies within the olecranon fossa may produce similar symptoms in the absence of osteophytic change.

Clinically there is often a history of repetitive hyperextension movements of the elbow.

The condition can be clinically demonstrated by extension of the elbow at which point a gentle hyperextension force is applied to the forearm (**Figure 12**). This will reproduce the patient's pain.

Anterior impingement occurs most commonly due to osteophytes on the coronoid process impinging into the coronoid fossa. Occasionally anterior

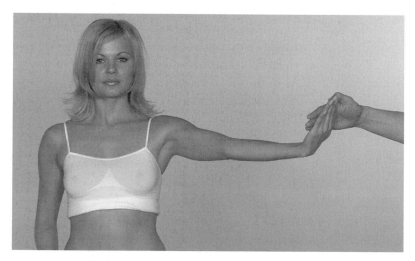

Figure 11 Provocation testing for medial epicondylitis.

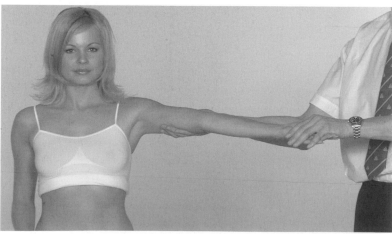

Figure 12 Impingement testing. Hyperextension of the elbow causes pain.

impingement is the result of osteophytic change within the radial fossa such that on full flexion the radial head impinges with the osteophytes.

Instability of the elbow

Varus instability

The lateral collateral ligament consists of the radial collateral ligament and the lateral ulnar collateral ligament.

In order to assess varus instability the elbow should be flexed to approximately 30° in order to unlock the olecranon from its fossa. In addition this manoeuvre relaxes the anterior capsule. Varus stress is then applied across the elbow joint with the humerus in full internal rotation.[13] In the presence of varus instability the gap between the capitellum and radial head will increase (**Figure 13**). This can often be appreciated by clinical examination but can more easily be confirmed if the procedure is undertaken under image intensification. The elbow under examination should be compared with the normal side.

Valgus instability

Valgus instability is most commonly seen in throwing athletes. Assessment of the ulnar collateral ligament is best undertaken with the patient seated and the patient's forearm held securely between the examiner's arm and trunk. The patient's elbow is flexed to approximately 30° to unlock the olecranon from its fossa and then the ulnar collateral ligament is palpated whilst a valgus stress is applied to the elbow. Opening of the elbow, local pain and tenderness are compatible with an ulnar collateral ligament injury.[13]

Tears in continuity without gross instability can be assessed by the method described by O'Brien.[14] This involves holding the patient's thumb and fully flexing the elbow whilst a valgus stress is applied to the elbow joint (**Figure 14**).

Rotatory instability

Postero-lateral rotatory instability results from insufficiency of the lateral collateral ligament.

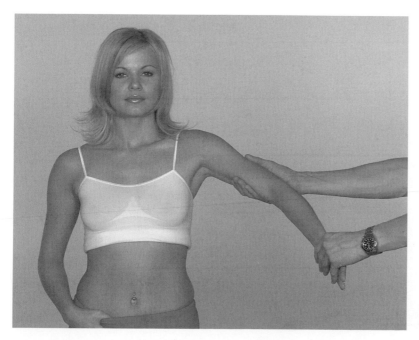

Figure 13 Varus instability testing. Varus stress is applied across the elbow with the humerus in full external rotation. If instability is present the gap between the capitellum and radial head increases.

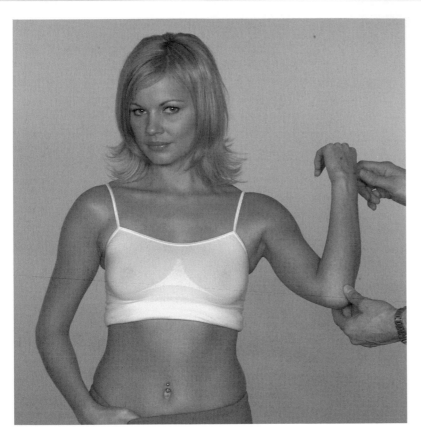

Figure 14 The milking test described by O'Brien for ulnar collateral ligament injuries in continuity without gross instability. A valgus stress is applied by pulling on the thumb whilst the elbow is fully flexed. If positive pain is experienced on full flexion of the elbow.

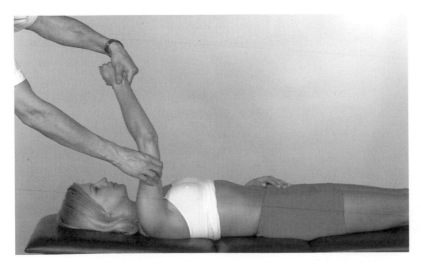

Figure 15 The lateral pivot shift test. With the patient lying supine and the arm above the head and forearm supinated a valgus force with axial compression is applied to the elbow. Subluxation produces a prominence over the radial head and a dimple in the skin behind it. Further extension causes a reduction to occur with a palpable, audible, clunk.

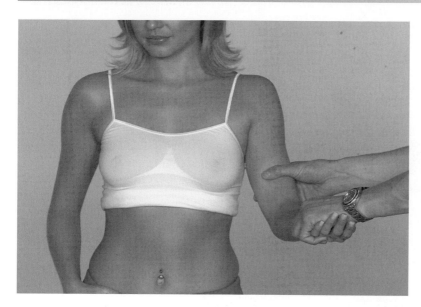

Figure 16 The postero-lateral rotatory drawer test. The elbow is flexed to 90° and the forearm fully supinated. The lateral forearm is grasped and an antero-posterior translation force applied. If positive instability is perceived by both the examiner and patient. The test is repeated at 30° of flexion.

The most sensitive clinical method of assessing insufficiency of the lateral collateral ligament is the lateral pivot shift test (**Figure 15**). The patient is positioned supine with the shoulder and elbow flexed to 90°. The patient's forearm is fully supinated and the examiner holds the patient's wrist and forearm and slowly extends the elbow whilst applying a valgus and axial compression force. This will often reproduce the patient's symptoms and give rise to apprehension. Subluxation of the radius and ulna from the humerus causes a prominence postero-laterally over the radial head and a dimple between the radial head and the capitellum. When the elbow is at approximately 40° of flexion the ulna suddenly reduces with a palpable and visible clunk.[15]

Postero-lateral rotatory draw test

This test may demonstrate subtle postero-lateral rotatory instability.

The elbow is flexed to 90° and the forearm is fully supinated. The lateral forearm is grasped and an antero-posterior translation force is applied (**Figure 16**). The lateral forearm pivots around the intact medial side. If the test results in a sense of instability perceived by both the examiner and the patient it is considered to be positive.[16] The test is repeated at 30° of flexion.

Apprehension signs

Asking a patient to rise from a chair using their arms to push them into the standing position may reproduce symptoms of instability. In such a situation the patient is reluctant to fully extend the elbow since the manoeuvre involves an axial load, valgus and supination of the forearm. A similar situation occurs if the patient is asked to perform a press-up. The same forces are applied to the elbow and once more result in apprehension.[17] The patient is reluctant to fully extend the elbow (**Figure 17**).

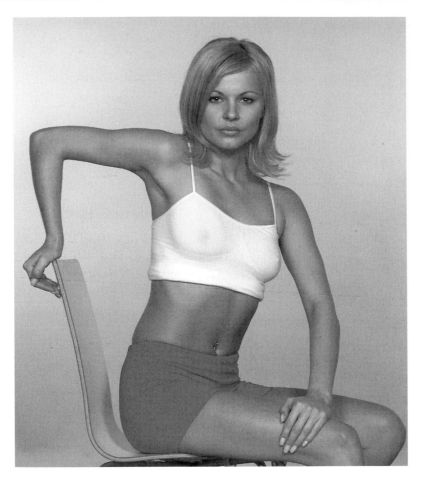

Figure 17 Apprehension signs. The patient is reluctant to fully extend the elbow when rising from a chair and pushing up with their arms.

References

1. Andrews JR, Whiteside JA. Common elbow problems in the athlete. *Journal of Orthopaedic Sports Physiotherapy* 1993; **6:** 289–95

2. Stanley D. Prevalence and aetiology of symptomatic elbow osteoarthritis. *Journal of Shoulder and Elbow Surgery* 1994; **3:** 386–9

3. Major HP. Lawn Tennis Elbow. *BMJ* 1883; **2:** 557

4. Mardam-Bey T, Ger E. Congenital radial head dislocation. *Journal of Hand Surgery* 1979; **4:** 316–20

5. Thompson H, Garcia A. Myositis ossificans: aftermath of elbow injuries. *Clinical Orthopaedics* 1967; **50:** 129–34

6. Baker BE, Bierwagen D. Rupture of the distal tendon of biceps brachii. *Journal of Bone and Joint Surgery* 1985; **67A:** 414–7

7. Hartz CR, Linscheid RL, Gramse RR, Daube JR. The pronator teres syndrome: compressive neuropathy of the median nerve. *Journal of Bone and Joint Surgery* 1981; **63A:** 885–90

8. Spinner M, Kaplan EP. The relationship of the ulnar nerve to the medial intermuscular septum in the arm and it's clinical significance. *Hand* 1976; **8:** 239–42

9. Bennett BS. Triceps tendon rupture. *Journal of Bone and Joint Surgery* 1962; **44A:** 741–4

10. Morrey BF, Chow EY. Passive motion of the elbow joint. *Journal of Bone and Joint Surgery* 1976; **58A:** 501–8

11. Yamamoto I, Ishii S, Usui M, Ogino T, Kaneda K. Cubitus varus deformity following supracondylar fracture of the humerus: a method for measuring rotational deformity. *Clinical Orthopaedics* 1985; **201:** 179–85

12. Nirschl RP. Elbow tendinosis / tennis elbow. *Clinical Sports Medicine* 1992; **4:** 851–70

13. Regan WD, Korinek SL, Morrey BF, An KN. Biomechanical study of ligaments about the elbow joint. *Clinical Orthopaedics* 1991; **271:** 271-

14. Jobe F, Elattrache N. Reconstruction of the MCL. In Morrey BF (ed): *Masters Techniques: The Elbow.* Philadelphia, Raven Press 1994

15. O'Driscoll SW, Bell DF, Morrey BF. Postero-lateral rotatory instability of the elbow. *Journal of Bone and Joint Surgery* 1991; **73A:** 440–6

16. Morrey BF, O'Driscoll SW. Lateral Collateral Ligament Injury. In Morrey BF (ed): *The Elbow and its Disorders* – Third Edition. Philadelphia, WB Saunders Company, 2000

17. Regan WD, Morrey BF. Physical Examination of the Elbow. In Morrey B F (ed): *The Elbow and its Disorders* – Third Edition. Philadelphia, WB Saunders Company, 2000

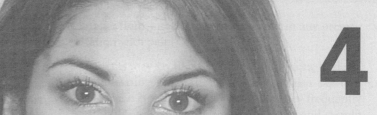

4

Examination of Peripheral Nerves in the Hand and Upper Limb

J Srinivasan & L C Bainbridge

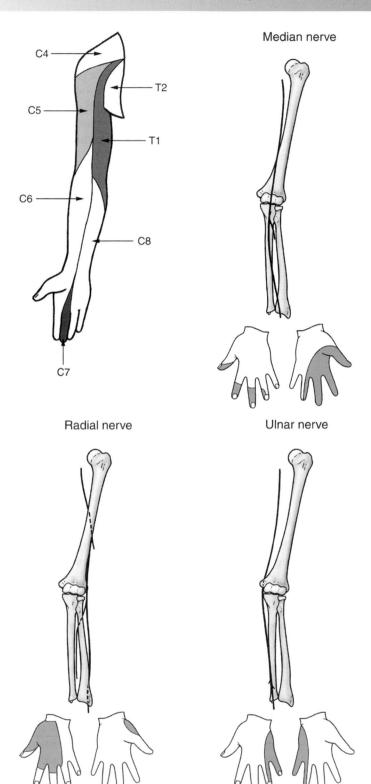

Median nerve

Radial nerve

Ulnar nerve

Figure 1 Diagram showing the dermatomes of the upper limb and territories of the peripheral nerves.

possible nerve damage. A deep laceration over the distal wrist with definite damage to the palmaris longus tendon will immediately raise the possibility of median nerve injury.

General

Warmth and sweating should be compared with the normal side. The 'Tactile adherence test[3] is useful to assess sweating in digits. This can be performed by sliding a smooth object (e.g. ball point pen) over the area of skin to be tested. A normal sweating pattern will impart some resistance to this movement: on a dry, denervated digit the pen slides freely. In patients who are unconscious or uncooperative and in children, a similar assessment can be done using the "skin wrinkling test"[4] – the affected finger or hand is immersed in warm water for 5–10 minutes. Denervated skin will not show a normal wrinkling pattern on the pulp. This test is also useful for monitoring nerve recovery in patients or detecting malingering.

Touch sensation should be compared on both sides of the digit and both hands should be assessed. Examination of the 'autonomous' areas of specific nerves will give more reliable information in proximal nerve injuries (*see* **Figure 1**). However the examination of touch sensation can be difficult to assess. A good examiner will certainly be able to differentiate between digital nerve injuries with some accuracy but even isolated dorsal branch injuries should be identified. The technique for examination is vitally important. Sharp implements such as pins and hypodermic needles, even if blunted, have **NO** place in the examination of touch and should only be used by neurologists. Touch should be evaluated by the use of pieces of cotton wool or simply using the examiner's own fingers. Initial evaluation in unilateral conditions should be made by comparing the two sides. Both sides are touched simultaneously and the patient is asked to compare the two sensations. In bilateral conditions the comparison should be between affected and unaffected areas. Progressively the areas examined are refined, from fingers on both hands to fingers on the same hand but different nerve territories to defined areas on the same finger comparing the radial and ulnar pulp in the case of a digital nerve injury in the finger.

Tinel's sign is one of the most important tests in evaluation of peripheral nerves. Light percussion along the course of the nerve from distal to proximal direction will elicit sharp pain over the recovering nerve fibres and paresthesiae along the course of the nerve. The alternative test is to start proximally in normal tissue and percuss in a distal direction until paraesthesia and sharp pain are elicited. This will usually be at the most proximal site of injury. A progressive advancement of the distal Tinel down the arm indicates recovery. Alternatively a static Tinel's indicates failure to recover and is a strong indicator for reassessment of the treatment strategy, perhaps indicating re-exploration in the traumatic case.

"Objective" Clinical Tests

These tests serve only as an indication of nerve function not of the patient's level of disability. We group these tests to assess 3 categories of clinical conditions:

1. **Acute injury**
   - Tactile adherence test
   - Assessment of touch sensation
   - Skin wrinkling
   - Electrical resistance

2. **Chronic conditions**
   - Static and moving two point discrimination
   - Semmes-Weinstein monofilaments
   - Pin wheel testing

2. **Assessment of recovery**
   - Static and moving two point discrimination
   - Semmes-Weinstein monofilaments
   - Skin wrinkling
   - Tactile adherence test

1. Static and moving two point discrimination are the most commonly used, so called 'objective tests'. They assess the innervation density of the slow and fast adapting receptors in the skin.[5,6] The results are unreliable in those with calloused hands. It is important to remember that the points should be applied with just less than the force required to blanch the skin at the points. The normal values for 2PD become progressively wider from distal to proximal – 4–5 mm in distal phalanx as against 20–50 mm

in forearm. Both can be assessed with a bent paperclip but preferably with a specialist device, e.g. Vernier calliper or the Disk-criminator. Moving two-point discrimination will usually be noted first in nerve recovery.

2. Semmes – Weinstein monofilaments assess the threshold of the slow adapting fibres. The levels are mapped out by using progressively thinner filaments.

3. The 'pin prick' test is employed occasionally to assess return of 'protective sensation' after nerve injury. However, it is uncomfortable to the patient and best avoided. Testing with a pinwheel is relatively patient-friendly and always performed from normal to abnormal areas.

Investigations

Neurophysiological tests are considered by many to be the 'gold standard' in peripheral nerve evaluation. After experimental median nerve compression, Gelberman noted a decrease in sensory amplitude to be the first abnormality. However we have to remember that the diagnosis of most nerve compression syndromes is a clinical one and that nerve conduction studies can confirm but cannot exclude intermittent or mild nerve compression. Nerve conduction study (NCS) and electromyography (EMG) can also help to identify neurapraxia from axonotmesis – a very useful differentiation in clinical management. Neurapraxia, where axonal continuity is preserved, should show full recovery within one to four months, regardless of the level of injury. On the contrary, recovery after axonotmesis depends on the level of injury and may take 4 to 18 months.

Skin resistance and conductance measurements have also been used in an effort to quantify the amount of sweating. However despite their proponents' quoted accuracy they have not achieved widespread acceptance.

Vibrometry assesses the thresholds of the faster adapting fibres and is usually assessed at two frequencies. Despite its claimed usefulness the equipment can be difficult to use and is still used mainly as a research tool except in assessment of Vibration White Finger.

Examination of specific nerves

Compression neuropathy and traumatic injury are the two main causes of peripheral nerve symptoms in the hand and elbow. General evaluation of the injured nerve is outlined in the previous sections. Here specific tests and signs will be discussed for each of the three main nerves in forearm and hand.

Median nerve – at wrist

Carpal tunnel syndrome (CTS) is the most commonly recognised peripheral nerve compression. Diagnosis is essentially based on the history and clinical findings. Specific tests are:

1. Phalen's test[7] with the wrist maximally flexed. Reproduction of symptoms – paresthesiae, pain – within 30 to 60 seconds is strongly suggestive of median nerve compression (**Figure 2**).

2. Reverse Phalen's with the wrist maximally extended. Again reproduction of the symptoms is the end point.

3. McMurtry[8] described a method where direct pressure applied over the median nerve at the distal wrist crease level reproduced the symptoms within 30 seconds to 2 minutes. Unlike Phalen's test, there is no wrist movement involved in this test. This is very useful in patients with painful wrist conditions or wrist stiffness. In his modification, Durkan[9] advised that pressure should be applied using both thumbs over the carpal tunnel itself (**Figure 3**).

4. The most specific muscle to be tested for CTS is the Abductor Pollicis Brevis (APB) – the most radial of the muscles in the thenar eminence. Keeping the dorsum of the hand flat on the table, the patient is directed to raise/abduct the thumb towards the ceiling and maintain it against resistance. The muscle can be seen to contract in the unaffected situation. Any weakness of the affected side can be compared with unaffected side. Thenar muscle wasting will indicate severe and long-standing median nerve compression (**Figure 4**).

5. The palmar cutaneous branch of the median nerve is given off about 3–5 cm proximal to

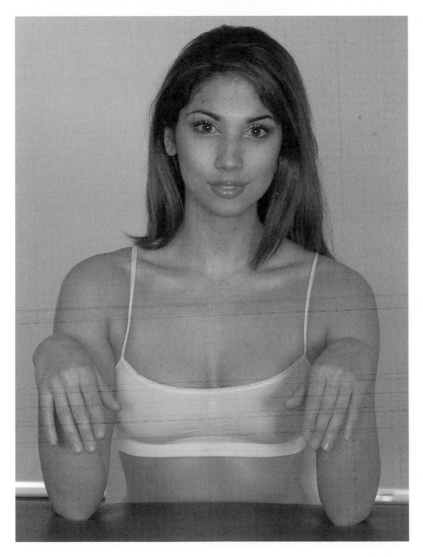

Figure 2 Phalen's test performed by resting the elbows on the desk and allowing the wrists to passively palmar flex with gravity.

wrist crease and runs above the level of transverse carpal ligament. Consequently, in a classical CTS, normal sensation is expected in the skin over Thenar eminence – numbness will indicate a proximal level nerve compression (e.g. Pronator Teres syndrome).

6. Other less common tests include the 'Tourniquet test'[10] and 'Straight Arm Raising' (SAR) test[11] – simply elevating the arm above the head level with wrist in neutral position may precipitate the symptoms of nerve compression by increasing the nerve ischaemia.

Median nerve – at proximal forearm and elbow

Factors responsible for proximal nerve compression are, from proximal to distal:

1. *Ligament of Struthers*: This is an aberrant ligament which when present is found to lie between the medial epicondyle of the humerus and a bony spur located 5 cm proximally on the humeral shaft. The Median nerve along with the brachial artery and vein run between the ligament and the humerus where it is liable to compression (**Figure 5**).

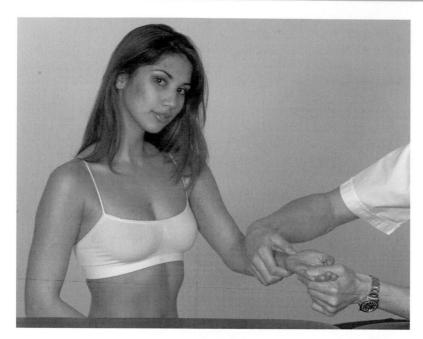

Figure 3 McMurtry's Test. The examiner applies pressure with the thumb over the volar aspect of the wrist reproducing the symptoms of median nerve entrapment.

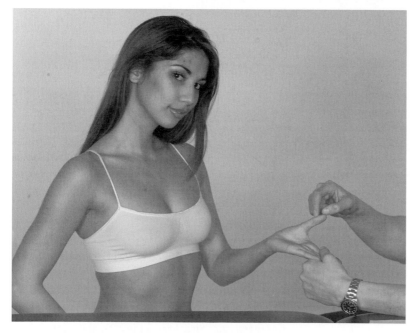

Figure 4 Resisted abduction of the thumb. The abductor pollicis brevis is the most radial of the thenar muscles and can be seen and felt to contract.

2. *Pronator syndrome*: Along its course from the elbow into the forearm the Median nerve runs beneath the thick lacertus fibrosus (extending from biceps tendon to the forearm fascia); between the superficial and deep heads of Pronator Teres and beneath the fibrous arch of the Flexor digitorum superficicalis (FDS) muscle – any one or a combination of them are possible sources of compression.

Clinically, the patient may present with features of carpal tunnel compression – but in addition,

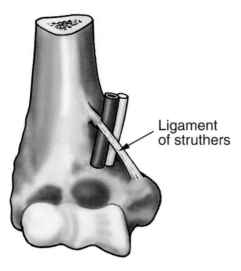

Figure 5 The Ligament of Struthers and its relationship to the median nerve and brachial artery.

complain of other specific problems. As mentioned above, the skin over the Thenar eminence will be numb – an important point of differentiation from CTS. In addition patients will complain of a dull ache in proximal forearm accentuated by use.

Apart from general signs – Tinel's and direct pressure – some of the specific, provocative tests[12] to test all the potential sites of compression listed above are:

- The patient's elbow is flexed and forearm pronated. The patient is then instructed to supinate the forearm forcibly, against resistance. The biceps tendon and lacertus fibrosus become taut and may exacerbate the symptoms (**Figure 6**).

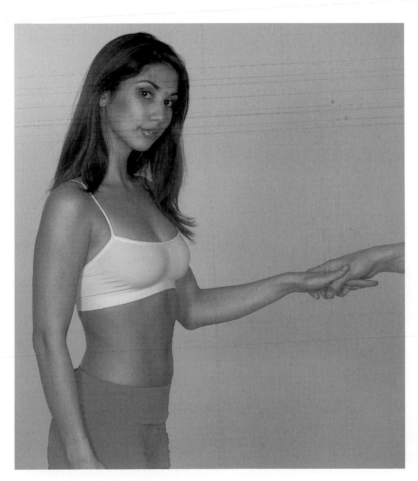

Figure 6 Resisted supination of the forearm which may result in compression of the median nerve through its effects on the lacertus fibrosus and biceps.

- The patients forearm is placed in full supination and the patient instructed to forcibly pronate the arm against resistance. This will tighten Pronator teres and increase any median nerve entrapment (**Figure 7**).

- Forceful flexion of the proximal interphalangeal joint of the middle finger against resistance will similarly increase any compression against the arch of the flexor digitorum superficialis (**Figure 8**).

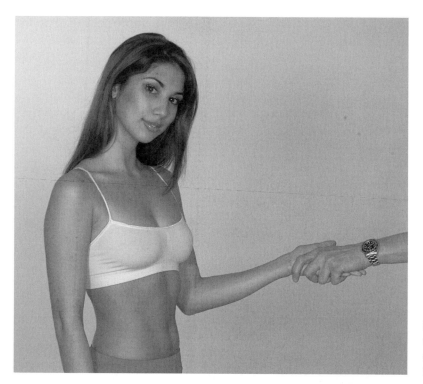

Figure 7 Resisted pronation which can also cause compression of the median nerve by the pronator teres.

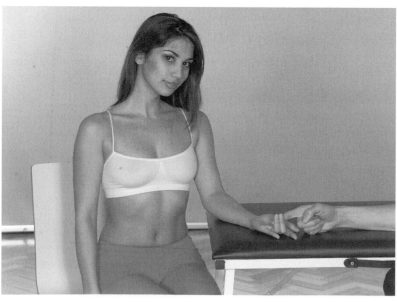

Figure 8 Resisted flexion at the PIPJ's of the middle and ring fingers which narrows the fibrous arch of the origin of the flexor digitorum superficialis which can also be a cause of median nerve entrapment at the elbow.

3. *Anterior interosseous syndrome*: The Anterior interosseous nerve is the last major motor branch of the Median nerve. It innervates Flexor Pollicis longus, Flexor digitorum profundus to the index and middle fingers as well as the Pronator Quadratus muscle. Isolated neuritis, as reported by Kiloh and Nevin,[13, 14] or compression by an abnormal band in Pronator teres or FDS muscle are common causes of these symptoms.

Clinically, loss of interphalangeal joint flexion of the thumb and the DIP joint of the index can be demonstrated. Instead of tip-to-tip pinch the so-called 'O' sign (**Figure 9**), the patient will only be able to make a side-to-side pinch.

Ulnar nerve – at elbow

The commonest site of ulnar nerve compression is in its course behind the medial epicondyle of the humerus – the 'cubital tunnel syndrome' (CUTS). Around this region, the nerve may be compressed by any of the following structures:

- The arcade of Struthers – a fascial band extending from medial intermuscular septum to the medial head of triceps.
- The medial intermuscular septum itself.[15]
- Exostoses from the medial epicondyle.
- The cubital tunnel and Osbourne's fascia – a fascial band bridging the two heads of flexor carpi ulnaris muscle.
- Accessory muscle – anconeus epitrochlearis

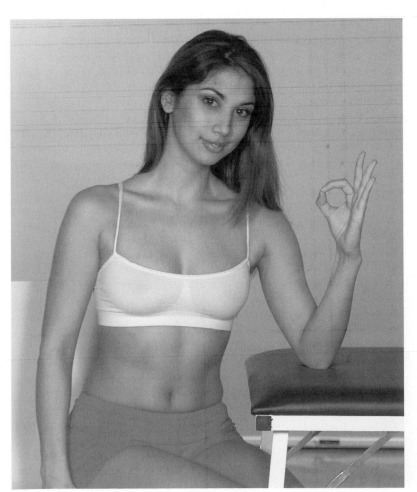

Figure 9 The Kiloh-Nevin sign assesses the intergrity of the anterior interosseous nerve. If the FPL and FDP to the index are intact and working the patient should be able to make an 'O'. If not only the pulps of the finger and thumb can be approximated rather than the tips.

Direct compression over the relevant pressure point will reproduce the clinical symptoms of paresthesiae over the ulnar border of the hand and Tinel's will also usually be positive over the relevant point.

Specific provocation tests are:

1. Elbow flexion test[16] – the patient is asked to supinate and flex the elbow fully. Hyperextension of the wrist in this position, for 3-5 minutes, is said to exacerbate the symptoms in cubital tunnel syndrome. Addition of 90 degrees of shoulder abduction to this posture may also increase the positive yield (**Figure 10**).

Long-standing ulnar nerve compression will result in intrinsic muscle weakness in the hand.

1. The patient may notice *clawing* of the little and ring fingers. The index and middle fingers are less affected as the first two lumbricals are innervated by median nerve. Unlike any other peripheral nerve lesions, the claw deformity is more pronounced with **distal** ulnar nerve lesions as the deep flexors, which are partly responsible for the clawing are innervated in the proximal forearm – the 'ulnar paradox'.

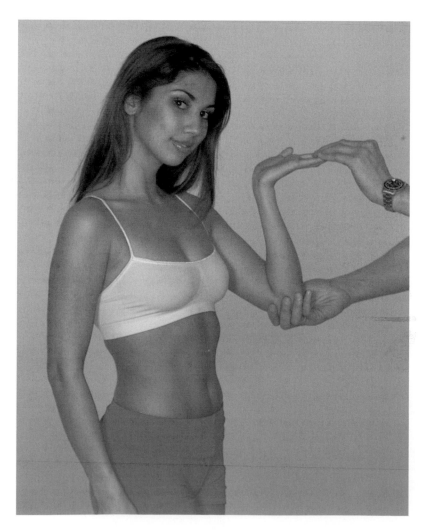

Figure 10 The elbow flexion test. The elbow is maximally flexed and supinated with the wrist hyper-extended. This is a provocative test for ulnar nerve entrapment at the elbow.

2. *Froment's sign*: direct the patient to grasp a card between the thumb and index finger in the first web space. The examiner then attempts to pull the card from between the finger and thumb. The weak adductor pollicis and first dorsal interosseous muscles will not be able to apply pressure to resist and the FPL will come into action leading to flexion of the IPJ of the thumb (**Figure 11**).

3. *Wartenburg sign*: This is considered as one of the earliest signs. The little finger will adopt an abducted posture – due to the weakness of the third palmar interosseus muscle (**Figure 12**)

4. *"Making a wish" sign*: The patient will be unable to cross his index finger over the middle finger due to the weakness of the intrinsics.

Ulnar nerve – at wrist (ulnar tunnel syndrome)[17]

From the forearm, the ulnar nerve enters the hand through Guyon's canal – with the pisiform lying ulnarly and then the hook of Hamate radially. Compression in this region may be due to irritation from an arthritic piso-triquetral joint, fracture of the hook of hamate or due to repeated trauma over the hypothenar area – the latter may present with thrombosis of the ulnar artery as well – often described as 'Hypothenar hammer syndrome'.[18] The patient may exhibit pure motor weakness or a mixed presentation depending on the site of compression. If the hook of hamate is fractured then the deeper motor branch winding around it may become entrapped leading to a pure motor lesion. However, a predominantly sensory problem is seen more frequently.

Normal sensation over the dorsum of fourth and fifth metacarpals will differentiate the ulnar nerve compression at wrist (where the dorsal sensory branch has been spared) from cubital tunnel syndrome.

Martin – Gruber anastomosis[19]

Contrary to the popular teaching, the innervation pattern in the hand and forearm is not sacrosanct. Crossover of nerve fibres between the three major nerves in upper limb is possible. The most common exchange of fibres between median and ulnar nerve in the forearm is the Martin-Gruber anastomosis – allegedly present in about 15–20% of individuals. Here, motor fibres from median nerve cross over to the ulnar nerve in the proximal forearm. Clinically, this becomes significant, as normal intrinsic muscle function may exist in spite of the ulnar nerve being injured above the level of the anastomosis. A similar sharing of sensory fibres in the hand between these two nerves is also reported (Riche-Cannieu anastomosis).

Radial nerve compression – forearm

Radial nerve compression may be above the elbow (in the axilla or in the spiral groove of the humerus) or below the elbow. Only the latter is discussed here. Compression at or below the elbow usually presents as one of two entities: radial sensory nerve compression or posterior interosseous nerve compression.

Posterior interosseous syndrome

The posterior interosseous nerve represents the motor branch of the radial nerve. It passes into the forearm between the two heads of the supinator (the radial tunnel). The proximal boundary of the supinator is thickened and termed the – the arcade of Frohse.[20] This thickening can be the source of compression of the nerve. Patients may complain of pain over the lateral aspect of the elbow radiating into the forearm. It is important to distinguish this from lateral epicondylitis. In lateral epicondylitis the point of maximum tenderness is around the origin of the extensor carpi radialis brevis (ECRB). This is just anterior to the lateral epicondyle. In posterior interosseous syndrome pain is often provoked by applying pressure over the radial tunnel behind the mobile wad of three.[21] Severe compression of the posterior interosseous nerve results in motor deficits with loss of metacarpophalangeal joint extension of the fingers and loss of thumb extension. Loss of function of the extensor carpi ulnaris can also occur resulting in radial deviation of the wrist on extension. The reason for this is that the extensor carpi radialis longus is innervated by the radial nerve and the extensor carpi radialis brevis by

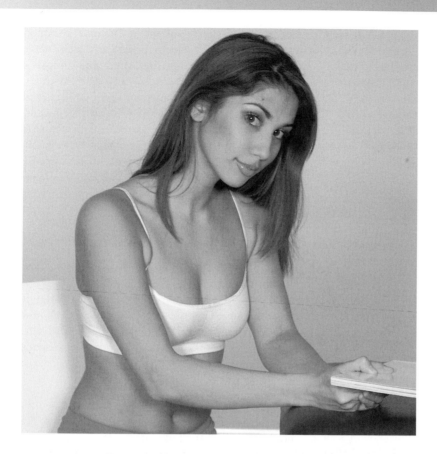

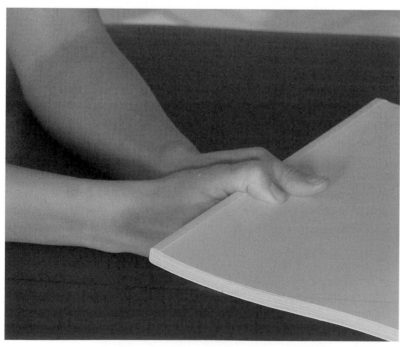

Figure 11 Froment's sign. Weakness of the intrinsics leads to the recruitment of the long flexor of the thumb.

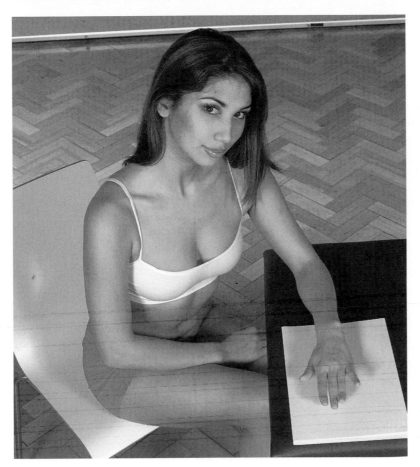

Figure 12 Wartenburg's sign. Abduction of the little finger is a sign of an ulnar nerve lesion due to weakness of the 3rd palmar interosseous muscle.

the posterior interosseous nerve proximal to the radial tunnel (its last branch before it enters the radial tunnel). These are always spared therefore in radial tunnel syndrome. The extensor carpi ulnaris however is innervated in the forearm distal to the tunnel.

A specific, provocative test is:

- *Resisted active supination* with the elbow in extension will increase the pressure beneath the Arcade of Froshe – this will increase the pain if the posterior interosseous nerve is already being compressed (**Figure 13**).

Radial sensory nerve (RSN) compression at forearm

This terminal branch of the radial nerve emerges through the deep fascia at the level of the distal third of the forearm, after its course beneath the brachioradialis tendon. First described by Wartenburg[22] in 1932, this entrapment has also been reported after repeated trauma from watchband and handcuffs. Wrist pronation causes a scissoring action between the extensor tendons and brachioradialis tendon with the RSN caught between them. This commonly presents with localised tenderness, which must be differentiated from conditions such as DeQuervain's disease.

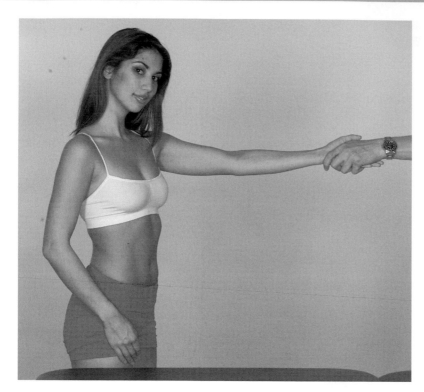

Figure 13 Resisted active supination of the forearm with the elbow in extension tightens the arcade of Frohse reproducing symptoms of posterior interosseous nerve entrapment.

References

1. Kaplan SJ, Glickel SZ, Eaton RG. Predictive factors in the non surgical treatment of carpal tunnel syndrome. *J Hand Surgery* (1990) **15B:** 106–108

2. Grossman LA, Kaplan JH, Downby FD, Grossman M. Carpal tunnel syndrome – initial manifestation of systemic disease. *JAMA* (1961) **176:** 259–261

3. Harrison SH. Tactile adherence test estimating loss of sensation after nerve injury. *Hand* (1974) **6:** 148–149.

4. O'Riain S. New and simple test of nerve function in hand. *BMJ* (1973) **3:** 615–616

5. Dellon AL, MacKinnon SE, Crosby PM. Reliability of two point discrimination measurements. *J Hand Surgery* (1987) **12:** 693–696

6. Gellis M, Pool R. Two point discrimination distances in the normal hand and forearm. *Plastic and Reconstructive Surgery* (1977) **59:** 58–63

7. Phalen GS. Spontaneous compression of the median nerve at the wrist. *JAMA* (1951) **145:** 1128–1131

8. Paley D, McMurtry R. Median nerve compression test in carpal tunnel syndrome diagnosis reproduces signs and symptoms in affected wrist. *Orthopaedic Review* (1985) **14:** 411

9. Durkan JA. A new diagnostic test for carpal tunnel syndrome. *J Bone and Joint Surgery* (1991) **73A:** 535–538

10. Gilliatt R, Wilson T. A pneumatic tourniquet test in the carpal tunnel syndrome. *Lancet* (1953) **2:** 595

11. Madan S, O'Connor D, Samuel AW. Efficacy of a new provocative test in the diagnosis of carpal tunnel syndrome: the Straight Arm Raise (SAR) test. Presented at BSSH Autumn meeting, Blackpool, UK. October 1999

12. Johnson RK, Spinner M, Shrewsbury MM. Median nerve entrapment syndrome in the proximal forearm. *J Hand Surgery* (1979) **4A:** 48–51

13. Kiloh LG, Nevin S. Isolated neuritis of Anterior Interosseus nerve. *BMJ* (1952) **1:** 850

14. Spinner M. The Anterior interosseus syndrome. *J Bone and Joint Surgery* (1970) **52A:** 84–94

15. Spinner M, Kaplan EB. The relationship of the ulnar nerve to the medial intermuscular septum in the arm and its clinical significance. *Hand* (1976) **8:** 239

16. Buelhler MJ, Thayer DT. The elbow flexion test. *Clinics of Orthopaedic Related Research* (1988) **233:** 213

17. Kleinert HE, Hayes JE. The ulnar tunnel syndrome. *Plastic and Reconstructive Surgery* (1971) **47:** 21

18. Conn J, Bergen JJ, Bell JL. Hypothenar hammer syndrome: post traumatic digital ischaemia. *Surgery* (1970) **68(6):** 1122–1128

19. Leibovic SJ, Hastings H. Martin-Gruber revisited. *J Hand Surgery* (1992) **17A:** 47

20. Spinner M. The arcade of Froshe and its relationship to posterior interosseus nerve paralysis. *J Bone and Joint Surgery* (1968) **50B:** 809

21. Sarhadi NS, Korday SN, Bainbridge LC. Radial tunnel syndrome: diagnosis and management. *J Hand Surgery* (1998) **23(5):** 617–619

22. Dellon AL, MacKinnon SE. Radial sensory nerve entrapment in the forearm. *J Hand Surgery* (1986) **11(2):** 199–205

Further Reading

Birch R, Bonney G, Wynn-Parry C B (Eds). *Surgical Disorders of the Peripheral Nerves.* Churchill Livingstone.

Dawson D, Hallett M, Millender L. *Entrapment neuropathies.* Little, Brown and Company.

Gelberman R (Ed). *Operative Nerve Repair and Reconstruction.* J B Lippincott Company.

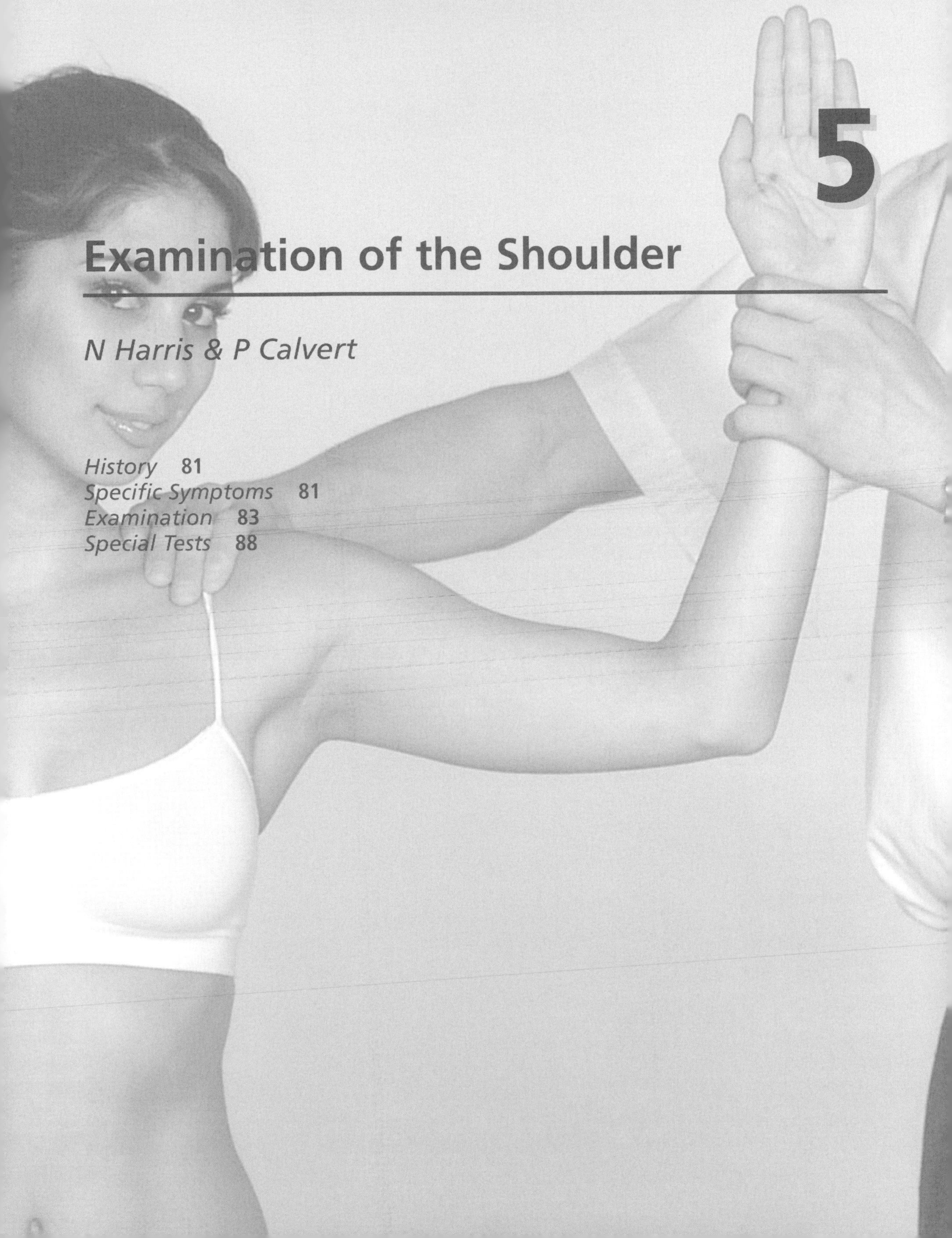

Examination of the Shoulder

N Harris & P Calvert

5

History

General

Important aspects in the general history of a patient with an apparent shoulder problem are age, handedness and occupation. Age alone will give a clue to diagnosis in that instability problems dominate in the second and third decades; impingement, frozen shoulder and inflammatory joint disease are mainly disorders of the fourth and fifth decades; beyond that rotator cuff tears and degenerative joint disease are more common. The main presenting complaint is usually pain, instability, weakness, stiffness, deformity or a combination. The duration of symptoms and whether the onset is related to a specific cause such as trauma or a change in occupation is relevant. How these symptoms interfere with activities of daily living, leisure and work must be recorded. A history of the previous treatments and the response to them should be documented. Enquiry is made about past medical history, general health and family history.

Specific Symptoms

Pain

Pain may be well localised or rather more diffuse. Pain from acromioclavicular joint pathology is usually well localised to that joint and the patient can often point to it with a single finger. ACJ pain may radiate more proximally to the root of the neck although this is not widely appreciated. Pain in the neck, over the trapezius or along the medial border of the scapula more commonly arises from the cervical spine. If it is associated with pain in the wrist or hand and certainly if paraesthesiae are present the cause is usually neurogenic, most often from the neck. It is possible, however, to get pain on the radial side of the wrist or hand and even into the thumb from intrinsic pathology in the shoulder. Poorly localised pain, particularly over the deltoid region commonly comes from subacromial and rotator cuff pathology. Night pain is frequently present with rotator cuff disease, glenohumeral arthritis and frozen shoulder. In young patients or if there are other suggestive signs or symptoms night pain should raise the suspicion of infection or tumour. Pain that radiates through to the back of the shoulder usually indicates glenohumeral pathology. Sudden onset of excruciating pain is typical of the resorptive phase of acute calcific tendonitis. This type of pain can be caused by acute brachial neuritis (Parsonage-Turner syndrome). With this diagnosis there is usually some associated weakness of shoulder girdle muscles which tends to be in a pattern not explicable on the basis of a single peripheral nerve or nerve root; for example scapula winging as well as weakness of only part of the deltoid may be seen.

Pain which occurs in part of the range of arm elevation is referred to as a painful arc. Pain which is worst in the midrange (e.g. 70 to 120) is typical of subacromial impingement and rotator cuff tendonitis whereas pain which is worst at the top of the range is typically caused by acromioclavicular joint disease. Frequently patients have a combination of these painful arcs. Pain related to the scapulothoracic joint can also cause a painful arc but the pain is felt posteriorly and might be associated with osteochondromas or bursitis.

Instability, catching and clicking

Instability is the symptomatic inability to maintain the humeral head centred in the glenoid. The use of an algorithm such as that described by Hawkins[1] is helpful in classification. **Figure 1** is the authors' modification of such a classification. TUBS (Traumatic, Unidirectional, Bankart, Surgery) and AMBRI (Atraumatic, Multidirectional, Bilateral, Rehabilitation, Inferior capsular shift) are useful "aide memoirs" for helping to differentiate between those likely to require surgery and those with a good chance of responding to a rehabilitation regime but it is not a comprehensive classification.[2] Events surrounding the initial episode must be clearly documented. If there was a history of trauma, enquiry should be made about the severity, the exact mechanism and whether the shoulder actually dislocated; if so what was the direction. The number of subsequent dislocations and the movements that precipitate them are noted. If there was no dislocation then

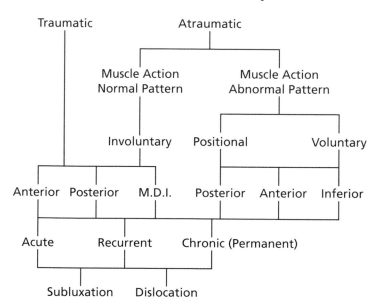

Classification of Instability

Figure 1 Algorithm to classify instability.

a careful history may well elicit clear evidence of subluxation. Rowe[3] describes the dead arm syndrome associated with anterior subluxation. It is worth noting that instability in the young patient can present as pain precipitated by provocative movements rather than definite episodes of dislocation or subluxation. If there was no history of trauma it is very important to ask if the patient can voluntarily dislocate the shoulder and whether it comes out every time the arm is in a specific position; the latter is suggestive of involuntary positional instability.[4] Finally, in patients with atraumatic instability, questions regarding generalised ligamentous laxity are included.

Painless clicks in the shoulder are common and may have no pathological significance. Painful clicks or catches can arise from the subacromial region but if felt deep inside the shoulder can be caused by labral tears. A SLAP lesion (superior labrum anterior to posterior (tear)) is difficult to diagnose clinically but is an example of a labral tear which may cause pain: it is most often found in throwing athletes.

Weakness

Weakness around the shoulder is the result of either intrinsic problems with the rotator cuff or neuromuscular problems such as cervical radiculopathy, brachial plexus injuries, entrapment of the suprascapular nerve or muscular dystrophy. In patients with suspected cuff pathology it is important to know whether the shoulder weakness followed a single traumatic event, suggesting an acute tear, or was of gradual onset indicative of an attrition rupture most likely secondary to impingement or intrinsic cuff degeneration. If weakness follows an injury to the shoulder then it is also important to consider neurological injury to the brachial plexus, particularly the axillary or suprascapular nerves; the combination of a rotator cuff tear with a nerve injury is often only partially diagnosed. Patients often describe the shoulder as being weak or stiff when movement is limited by pain. When it comes to examination, if this is suspected, it is important to abolish pain with local anaesthetic injections before assessing power. A history of neck pain and stiffness may help identify those patients with weakness secondary to nerve root compromise. Brachial plexus injuries are the result of violent blunt trauma to the head and neck, penetrating injuries to the posterior triangle of the neck or birth injuries and should be fairly obvious. A family history of shoulder weakness occurring bilaterally starting in early adulthood and associated with facial weakness is typical of facioscapulohumeral dystrophy. Patients complain of an inability to maintain their arms in an elevated position for long peroids. Suprascapular nerve entrapment is associated with diffuse posterolateral shoulder pain and weakness of abduction and external rotation.[5] Confirmation requires electromyographic studies.

Stiffness

A restriction of both active and passive shoulder movement may be caused by such disorders as frozen shoulder, osteoarthritis, rheumatoid arthritis and chronic dislocation. Patients with a primary frozen shoulder are most commonly in the fourth and fifth decades, more often female and usually present with a vague history of pain referred to the deltoid for several weeks or months followed by increasing pain and stiffness which progressively interferes with their activities of daily living. Diabetes mellitus is associated with primary frozen shoulder and patients with

diabetes have a less good prognosis for spontaneous recovery which takes longer. Other systemic disorders such as thyroid dysfunction are also associated with a frozen shoulder.

Frozen shoulder can be primary or secondary. Secondary frozen shoulder is a term, which should probably be abandoned and is better described as secondary stiffness; it can be the result of intrinsic problems related to the cuff or extrinsic problems such as humeral fracture or post-operative. Osteoarthritis may present in a similar way to a frozen shoulder but radiographs will differentiate. Patients with rheumatoid arthritis often have shoulder involvement. The pattern of other joint involvement should make the diagnosis straightforward. Other rarer causes of a stiff shoulder include conditions such as synovial chondromatosis and tumours.

Examination

Inspection

Inspection should follow a systematic approach. The patient should be undressed to the waist. Modesty in the female should be preserved by using a strapless garment to cover the breasts. It is important to watch the ease or difficulty with which the patient gets undressed and this must correlate with

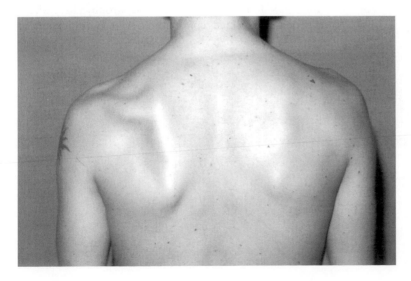

Figure 2 Example of severe infraspinatus wasting.

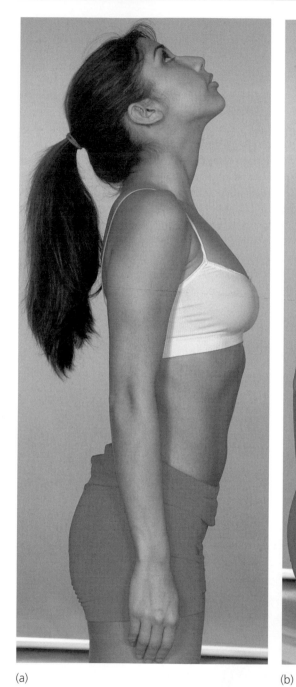

(a)

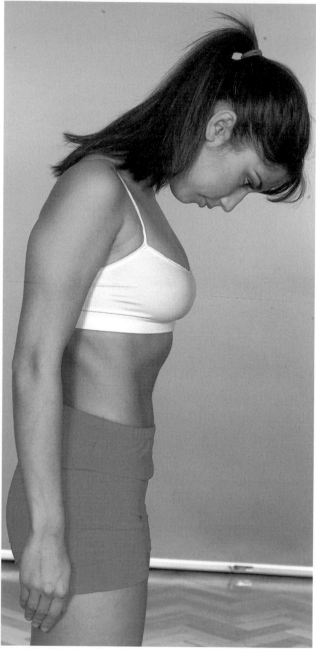

(b)

Figure 3 Cervical extension (a), flexion (b).

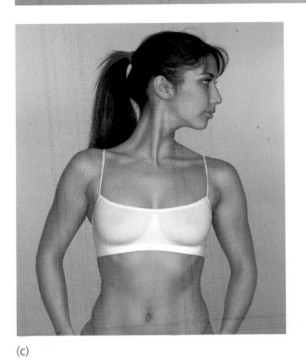

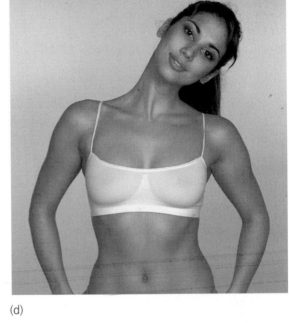

(c)

(d)

Figure 3 Lateral rotation (c), and lateral flexion (d).

the history. General appearance such as cachexia or pallor may indicate sinister underlying pathology. Scars from previous surgery or trauma should be documented. The patient must be inspected from the back as well as the front. Starting with the sternoclavicular joints medially any deformity or asymmetry suggestive of sternoclavicular pathology should be noted. The profiles of the clavicles and acromioclavicular joints should be compared. There may be evidence of a malunited fracture. Prominence of the acromioclavicular joint may be traumatic or degenerative. Squaring off of the shoulder profile may be related to wasting of the deltoid or medialisation of the humeral head as in erosive rheumatoid arthritis as well as to the more commonly appreciated anterior dislocation. The bulk of the pectoral and trapezius muscles should be compared on both sides. An abrupt "pop-eye" appearance of the biceps indicates rupture of the long head of biceps. Wasting of the cuff muscles in the supraspinous and infraspinous fossae is significant (**Figure 2**); it is most commonly caused by a

rotator cuff tear but neurological causes such as suprascapular nerve entrapment causing infraspinatus wasting should be considered. Winging of the scapulae and any asymmetry such as a high riding small scapula associated with a Sprengel shoulder is best assessed from the back. Winging can be caused by neurological lesions affecting the dorsal scapular, long thoracic or accessory nerves. Pseudowinging might be the result of a rib or scapular osteochondroma.

Palpation

Palpation should follow a systematic approach. Start with the sternoclavicular joint medially, move along the length of the clavicle to the acromioclavicular joint. Tenderness over the acromioclavicular joint is associated with degenerative change and traumatic subluxation. Occasionally a ganglion may be felt over the acromioclavicular joint with underlying degenerative changes. It is important to remember that degenerative change in the acromioclavicular

joint is part of the normal ageing process and is not necessarily the cause of symptoms. Tenderness along the anterior and anterolateral margin of the acromion is non-specific but may be associated with subacromial impingement. Palpation lateral and inferior to the coracoid might reveal tenderness typically associated with an inflammatory arthropathy or primary frozen shoulder whilst tenderness over the posterior joint line is more typical of osteoarthritis. Anteriorly palpation should continue distally. Approximately 7 cm distal to the acromion the examiner can palpate the region of the intertubercular sulcus. Tenderness here may reflect a bicipital tendonitis but it should be stated that localisation of tenderness is very non-specific for a particular diagnosis.

Movement

Both active and passive movement should be assessed. Before addressing the shoulder, the cervical spine should be examined to determine whether movement of the neck reproduces shoulder symptoms. In the fully extended cervical spine the nose parallels the floor and in the fully flexed position the patient should be able to get their chin on their chest.

Lateral rotation is approximately 80° and lateral flexion 40° (**Figure 3**).

Assessment of shoulder movement begins with forward elevation in the sagittal plane and abduction in the coronal plane. Elevation in the plane of the scapula can also be examined. The plane of the scapula is 20-30° forward of the coronal plane. The range of all these movements is 0-170° approximately but must be compared with the other side. External rotation is tested with the arm at the side and the elbow flexed to 90°. The normal range is 50-70°. External rotation can also be tested with the arm in 90° of abduction. The range is increased in this position and may be abnormally increased in throwing athletes. Internal rotation is assessed by noting the position reached by the extended thumb up the spine. The normal range is between T5-10 but again comparison must be made with the other side (**Figure 4**). The rhythm of shoulder movement is very important. This should be observed from behind.

The ratio of scapulothoracic to glenohumeral movement is usually 1:2. In the early stages of elevation movement occurs mainly, but not exclusively, in the glenohumeral joint. If, one wishes to quantify it the examiner stands behind the patient and fixes the tip of the scapula between index finger and thumb. The patient is then asked to elevate the arm. In the normal situation the arm can be abducted 80-90°. Further abduction is then restricted by the fixed scapula. When the scapula is released, further abduction is observed. In this way it is possible to distinguish between the glenohumeral and scapulothoracic components of abduction (**Figure 5**). The test can be repeated passively. Muscle testing will be discussed under special tests.

Neurovascular assessment

The general examination should always be completed with a brief assessment of the neurovascular status of both upper limbs. Sensation to light touch should be tested in dermatomes C4-T2. Power around the elbow, wrist and hand can then be assessed. Shoulder power will have been tested separately. Search should be made for specific patterns of peripheral nerve involvement, especially for injury to the axillary nerve. The biceps, brachialis and triceps reflexes complete a mini-neurological examination. Both radial pulses should be palpated.

Special Tests

Muscle testing

Testing deltoid function is best done with the arm in 90° of abduction and neutral rotation. With resistance the muscle can be seen and felt to contract. To assess supraspinatus function the "empty can" and "full can" tests have been described. In the empty can test desribed by Jobe and Moynes[6] the arm is abducted to 90°, then brought forward 30° into the plane of the scapula and then into maximal internal rotation (**Figure 6**). Muscle strength is then tested in this position. A modification to this described by Kelly et al[7] tests the supraspinatus in 45° of external rotation rather than in maximal internal rotation

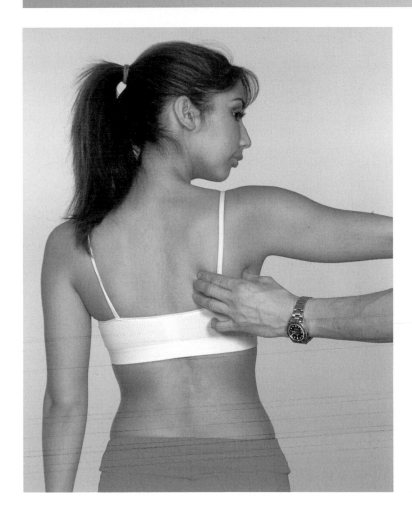

Figure 5 How to fix the scapula to differentiate between glenohumeral and scapulothoracic movement.

(**Figure 7**). Both are equivalent in terms of diagnostic accuracy but testing the supraspinatus in 45° of external rotation is less painful.[8] The external rotators, teres minor and infraspinatus, can be tested with the elbow at 90° and the arm by the side. The arm is passively maximally externally rotated and then released. If there is severe weakness of the external rotators then the arm will fall into internal rotation which Bigliani *et al* described as a "drop sign".[9] Hertel *et al*[10] described a modification of this sign which they termed the external rotation lag sign (ERLS). To elicit this sign the patient is seated with the examiner standing behind; the arm is supported at the elbow with that joint passively flexed to 90° and the shoulder elevated 20° in the scapula plane; the shoulder is placed in almost full external rotation by the examiner holding the wrist with his other hand. The patient is asked to maintain this position actively when the wrist is released. The sign is positive when there is a drop back towards neutral rotation (**Figure 8**). They also described a drop sign which differs from that described by Bigliani *et al.*[9] For this drop sign the arm is supported at the elbow with the shoulder elevated 90° in the scapular plane and almost fully externally rotated. Again the patient is asked to maintain this position when the examiner releases the wrist. The sign is positive if a lag or "drop" occurs (**Figure 9**). The inability to maintain the arm in an externally rotated position when bringing the hand to the mouth puts the arm

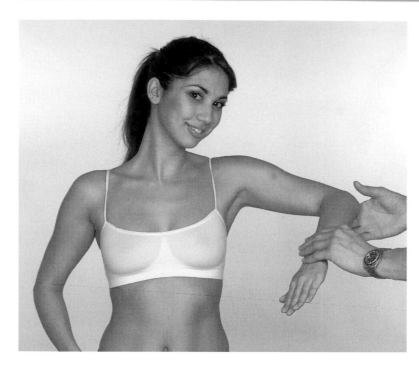

Figure 6 The "empty can test".

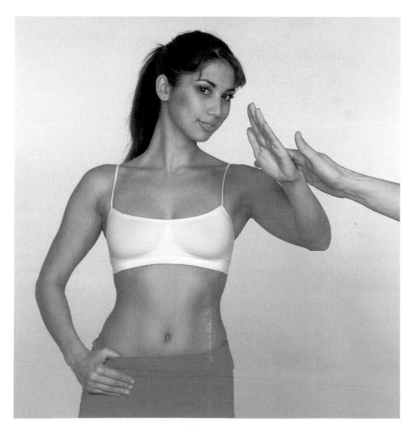

Figure 7 The "full can test".

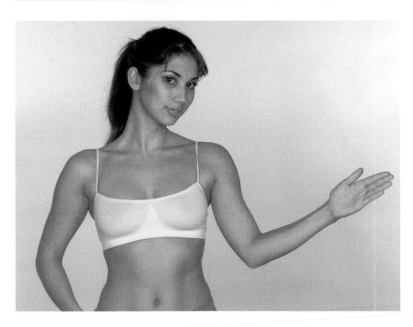

Figure 8 The external rotation lag sign (ERLS).

in a bugle position which has been termed the 'signe de clairon'.[11]

Gerber and Krushell described the lift off test for the assessment of subscapularis function.[12] The patient's shoulder is internally rotated and the dorsum of the hand placed over the lumbosacral junction. From this position the patient is asked to lift their hand off their back maximally extending and internally rotating the shoulder (**Figure 10**). Inability to do this suggests a subscapularis rupture. Hertel *et al*[10] described the internal rotation lag sign for the diagnosis of subscapularis ruptures and stated that it was as specific as the lift off test but more sensitive and had a greater negative predictive value because is could detect partial ruptures. The size of the angular lag correlated with the extent of the subscapularis rupture. In this test the elbow is passively flexed to 90° by the examiner and then the arm is maximally internally rotated and extended behind the back. The patient is asked to maintain this position. The sign is positive if lag occurs and the hand falls back towards the spine; the difference between the two sides can be used to quantify the findings (**Figure 11**). It should be noted that all the lag signs have limited use if the shoulder cannot be placed in the appropriate position either because of pain or limitation of passive movement.

Another technique to test subscapularis function is to ask the patient to place their hands on the abdomen. The examiner passively brings forward the elbows so they are anterior to the coronal plane of the body. The patient is asked to push their hands hard into their abdomen. If either arm falls behind the coronal plane of the body then this is suggestive of weakness of the subscapularis. This sign is called the "belly press test" or Napolean's sign (**Figure 12**). A further test the hug test has also been described by DeBeer (*personal communication*) and is thought to be particularly useful when assessing the subscapularis in cases of painful shoulders. The hand is placed across the front of the chest to reach the posterior axillary fold of the contra-lateral side. The patient squeezes their hand against their body and the examiner tries to pull it away. In a normal adult it should not be possible to pull the hand away from the body. Due to the extreme internal rotation it is felt that the pectoralis major does not play much of

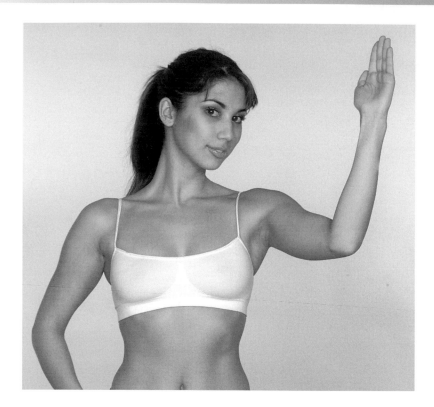

Figure 9 The "drop sign".

a roll and that subscapularis is relatively isolated. A spring loaded device can be used to measure strength and compare with the other side (**Figure 13**). The biceps can be tested using Yergasson's test with the arm at the side and the elbow flexed to 90°; the forearm is placed in full pronation and the patient attempts to supinate against resistance. Pain felt in the region of the bicipital groove is said to indicate bicipital tendonitis.[13] Speed's test has also been described to test the long head of biceps-superior labral complex. In this test the elbow is flexed to 30° with the forearm supinated and the patient asked to flex further against resistance; if shoulder pain is precipitated it is also said to suggest biceps tendonitis.[14] It is worth noting that all tests for bicipital tendonitis have a high sensitivity but low specificity.

In patients with facioscapulohumeral dystrophy the commonest complaint is of rapid fatigue when the arm is elevated. Copeland described standing behind the patient applying pressure over the scapula to prevent it winging. The patient is then asked to forward elevate to 90°. With the scapulothoracic joint held reduced the patient finds they are able to maintain this position longer.[15] A successful test is an indication the patient might benefit from a scapulothoracic fusion.

Impingement signs and tests

Neer[16] described his method for assessing subacromial impingement. In this the examiner stands behind the patient and the internally rotated arm is passively elevated in the scapular plane whilst stabilizing the scapula (**Figure 14**). Pain is usually elicited in the arc between 70 and 120°. Some pressure down onto the scapula at about 120° of elevation exacerbates the pain. The test is done by instilling local anaesthetic into the subacromial space and then repeating the manoeuvre used to elicit the sign. If the pain produced by the sign is abolished by the local anaesthetic that is a positive impingement test. Such a positive test is one of the best predictors of outcome of subacromial decompression. Various

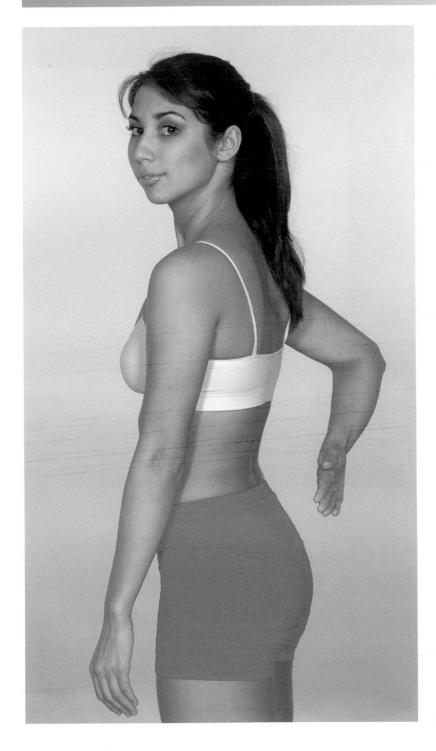

Figure 10 Gerber's lift-off test.

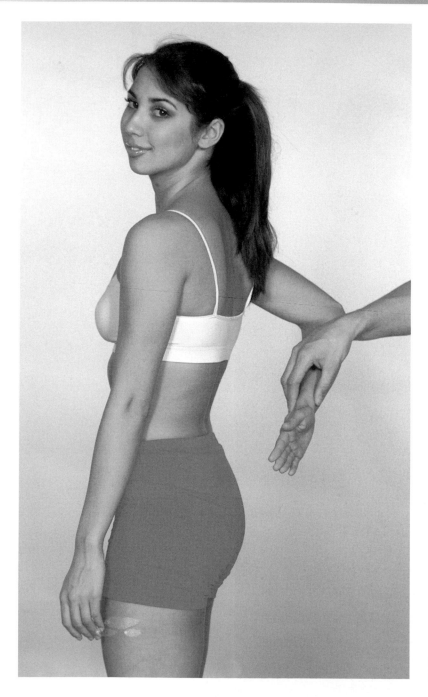

Figure 11 The internal rotation lag sign (IRLS).

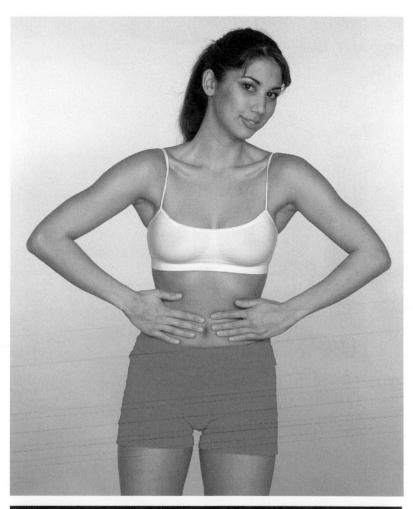

Figure 12 The "belly press test" (Napoleon's sign).

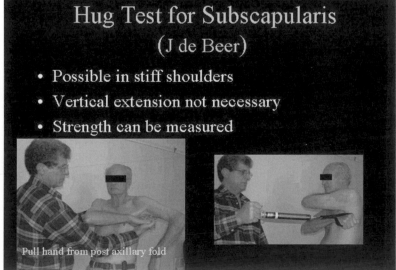

Hug Test for Subscapularis
(J de Beer)

- Possible in stiff shoulders
- Vertical extension not necessary
- Strength can be measured

Pull hand from post axillary fold

Figure 13 The "Hug Test".

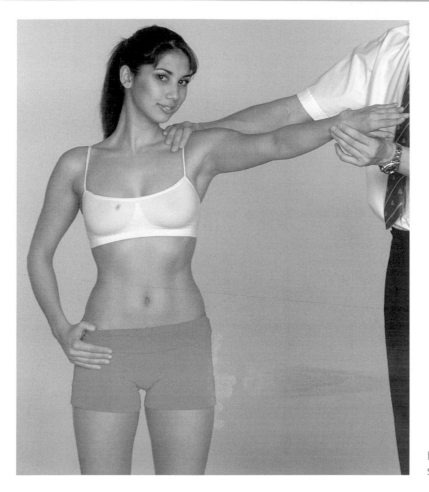

Figure 14 Neer's impingement sign.

modifications of this sign and test have been described but are all a variation on the theme. Hawkins and Kennedy[17] described their test with the arm elevated to 90° and adducted; the arm is then internally rotated maximally bringing the supraspinatus and greater tuberosity under the coracoacromial ligament and anteroinferior acromion; production of pain represents a positive test; this can also be repeated after injecting local anaesthetic into the subacromial space and resolution of the pain reinforces the diagnosis. The local anaesthetic will also abolish the midrange painful arc of elevation if it is caused by impingement. Great caution is required before diagnosing subacromial impingement in young patients; they should be closely evaluated for any evidence of instability,

which is most likely the primary cause of their impingement.

Acromioclavicular joint

Pain arising from the acromioclavicular joint can be reproduced at the top of the range of elevation. It is often necessary to ask the patient to elevate the arm to the maximum and for the examiner to then passively push it a little further in order to elicit the pain, which is well localised to the top of the shoulder in the region of the acromioclavicular joint. Acromioclavicular joint pain can also be tested by adduction of the arm across the chest. If the arm is forward flexed to 90° and then adducted to 15° with the hand in full pronation pain will be felt on top of the shoulder (**Figure 15**). In this position the greater tuberosity elevates the acromion locking and loading the acromioclavicular joint. The use of local anaesthetic testing is extremely useful for confirming that the pain elicited by these tests arises from the acromioclavicular joint. The joint is injected with one or two millilitres of local anaesthetic and the tests repeated. If the pain is abolished that is the best evidence that the acromioclavicular joint is the source.

Labral tears

These are difficult to diagnose clinically although various tests have been described. If the cross chest adduction manoeuvre used to test the acromioclavicular joint is repeated with with the hand in full supination the long head of biceps is tightened and the acromioclavicular joint relaxed by moving the greater tuberosity out of the way. If this manouvre causes pain, clicking, or catching felt inside the shoulder it is suggestive of a SLAP lesion.[18] Labral tears may be diagnosed using the crank test[19] but cuff tears, impingement and instability must be assessed first because they can produce similar findings with the test. The affected shoulder is passively elevated to 160° in the scapular plane, an axial load is applied along the humeral shaft whilst at the same time internally and externally rotating the arm. Pain, catching or clicking is suggestive of a labral tear. Snyder described a similar test but with the arm at 90° of abduction and compared it to McMurray's test for meniscal tears in the knee.[20]

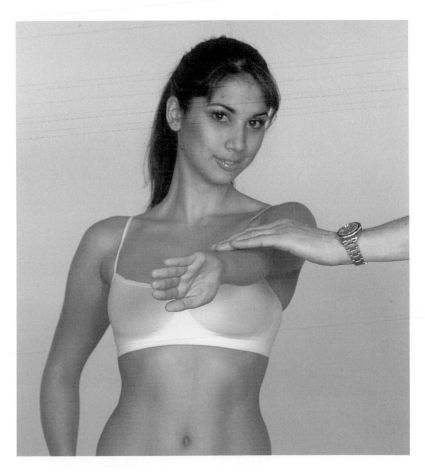

Figure 15 The "active compression test" to identify acromioclavicular impingement and labral tears.

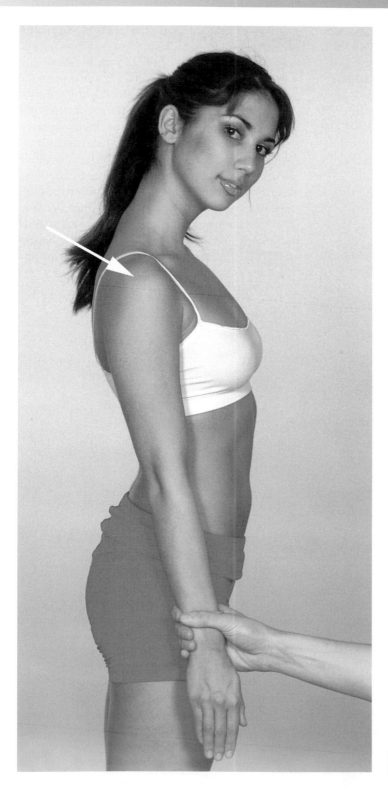

Figure 16 The sulcus sign indicative of inferior laxity.

Instability

Instability can be anterior, posterior or a combination of these. If there is an inferior component it has been classified as multidirectional. During the general examination features of generalised laxity such as hyperextension of the thumb, fingers, elbows and knees should be noted. Search for cutaneous manifestations of collagen disorders should be made; these may include thinning of the skin and widening of scars. Patients with anterior instability may also have a greater than average range of external rotation. Specific laxity tests are the sulcus sign and the anterior and posterior drawer tests or load and shift test. To demonstrate the sulcus sign inferior traction is applied to the arm. Gross instability is demonstrated by widening of the subacromial space more than 2 cm creating a sulcus distal to the lateral acromion (**Figure 16**). The anterior and posterior drawer tests are performed with the patient seated. The examiner stands behind the patient and holds the left scapula from above with the right hand with the thumb posteriorly and the middle finger on the coracoid; the index finger rests lightly on the anterior aspect of the humeral head to determine the degree of movement. The humeral head is held by the left hand between the thumb posteriorly and the index and middle fingers anteriorly. With the left hand the examiner firstly applies a load across the shoulder to ensure reduction and then applies anterior and posterior shearing forces. The amount of translation can be quantified by estimating the distance moved between the humeral head and coracoid (**Figure 17**).

Specific tests for instability are the anterior and posterior apprehension tests.

For the anterior apprehension test the examiner stands behind the patient with the palm of his contralateral hand stabilising the top of the scapula and the thumb resting on the posterior aspect of the humeral head. With his other hand he holds the patient's forearm and abducts the shoulder to 90° with the elbow flexed. Then at 90, 120 and 150 he extends and externally rotates the shoulder whilst maintaining gentle pressure with the thumb on the back of the humeral head. A positive apprehension test is when the pectoralis major contracts involun-

tarily, the patient resists the manoeuvre, gets an apprehensive look on the face and complains of their feeling of instability (Figure 18). Sometimes the patient just experiences pain with this test and in this circumstance or with equivocal apprehension the relocation test can help to distinguish pain caused by instability as opposed to other causes such as impingement. In this test, which must be conducted with the patient lying supine, the position of the arm for the anterior apprehension test is reproduced. The examiner then applies a posterior force at right angles to the shaft of the humerus. This should reduce the pain or feeling of apprehension if instability is the cause. When the posterior force is released or changed to an anterior pull the symptom returns. If impingement, either internal or external, is the cause then this manoeuvre should make no difference.

The posterior apprehension test is performed with the patient supine. The arm is maximally internally rotated and forward flexed to 90°. A posteriorly directed force is then applied to the humeral head by axial pressure along the humerus from the elbow (**Figure 19**). In a positive test the patient feels apprehensive and experiences the feeling of instability. The examiners other hand can be placed on top of the shoulder to assess the degree of subluxation. From this position the arm can be brought into abduction. The subluxed or dislocated humeral head should relocate during this manoeuvre.

Power

In order to complete a Constant score it is necessary to measure the power with the arm elevated to 90°. There has been considerable debate as to how this is best done and questions raised about its value and accuracy. In their original paper Constant and Murley described using a spring balance held by the patient with the arm elevated to 90° in the scapula plane.[21] A downward force is applied by the examiner to the spring balance until the patient is no longer able to maintain the elevated position. At that point the reading in pounds on the balance is noted and that is the value that should be entered in the power section of the Constant score. The test should be repeated to a total of three times and the average

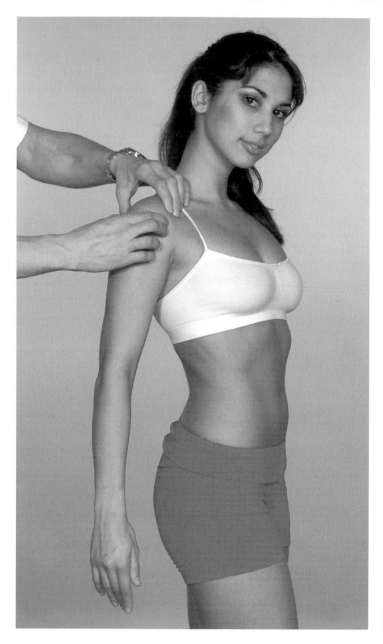

Figure 17 The anterior-posterior draw test.

used. It is perfectly acceptable to use something more sophisticated than a spring balance as the measuring device if it is available but the same position and principles should be applied and it should be supported from the patient's wrist (Figure 20).

Documentation

Finally having completed the examination it is important to record the findings clearly and accurately.

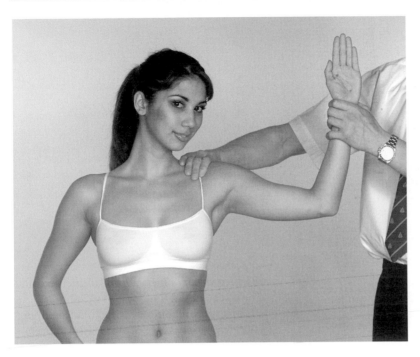

Figure 18 The anterior apprehension test.

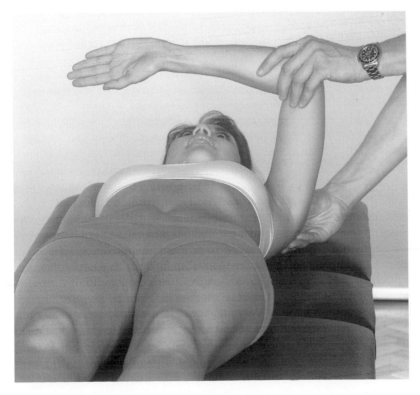

Figure 19 The posterior apprehension test.

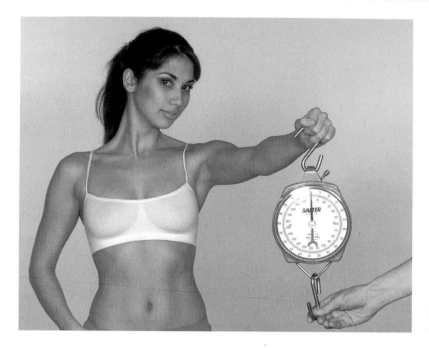

Figure 20 Power testing for a Constant score.

References

1. Silliman JF, Hawkms RJ. Classification and physical diagnosis of instability of the shoulder. *Clin Orth* 1993; **291:** 7–19

2. Thomas SC, Matsen FA. An approach to the repair of avulsion of the glenohumeral ligaments in the management of traumatic anterior glenohumeral instability. *J Bone Joint Surg* 1989; **71A:** 506–513

3. Rowe CR, Zarins B. Recurrent transient anterior subluxation of the shoulder. *J Bone Joint Surg* 1981; **63A:** 863–872

4. Involuntary positional instability of the shoulder in adolescents and young adults. Is there any benefit from treatment? Takwale VJ, Calvert P, Rattue H. *J Bone Joint Surg* 2000; **82B:** 719–723

5. Fabre Th, Piton C, Leclouerec G, Gervais-Delion F, Durandeau A. Entrapment of the suprascapular nerve. *J Bone Joint Surg* 1999; **81B(3):** 414–419

6. Jobe FW, Moynes DR. Delineation of diagnostic criteria and a rehabilitation program for rotator cuff injuries. *Am J Sports Mod* 1982; **10:** 336–339

7. Kelly BT, Kadrmas WR, Speer KP. The manual muscle examination for rotator cuff strength: An electromyographic investigation. *Am J Sports Mod* 1996; **24:** 581–588

8. 1toi E, Kido T, Sano A, Masakazu U, Sato K. Which is the more useful the "full can test" or the "empty can test", in detecting the torn supraspinatus tendon. *Am J Sports Med* 1999; **27(1):** 65–68

9. Bigliani LU, Cordasco FA, McIlveen SJ, Musso ES. Operative treatment of massive rotator cuff tears: long term results. *J Shoulder Elbow Surg* 1992; **1:** 120–30

10. Hertel R, Ballmer FT, Lambert SM, Gerber Ch. Lag signs in the diagnosis of rotator cuff rupture. *J Shoulder Elbow Surg* 1996; **5(4):** 307–313

11. Gerber C, Hersche 0. Tendon transfer for the treatment of irreparable rotator cuff defects. *Orthopaedic Clinics of North America* 1997; **28:** 195–204

12. Gerber C, Krushell RJ. Isolated tears of the subscapularis muscle. Clinical features in sixteen cases. *J Bone Joint Surg* 1991; **73B:** 389–99

13. Yergason RM. Supination sign. *J Bone Joint Surg* 1931; **13:** 160

14. Field LD, Savoie FH. Arthroscopic suture repair of superior labral detachment lesions of the shoulder. *American Journal of Sports Medicine* 1993; **21:** 783–791

15. Copeland SA, Howard RC. Thoracoscapular fusion for facioscapulohumeral dystrophy. *J Bone Joint Surg* 1978: **60(B):** 547–51

16. Neer CS II, Welsh PR. The shoulder in sports. *Orthop Clin North Am* 1977; **8:** 583–591

17. Hawkins RJ, Kennedy JC. Impingement syndromes in athletes. *Am J Sports Medicine* 1980; **8:** 151–157

18. O'Brien S, Pagnam MJ, Fealy S, McGlynn SR, Wilson JB. The active compression test: A new and effective test for diagnosing labral tears and acromioclavicular joint abnormality. *Am J Sports Medicine* 1998; **26(5):** 610–613

19. Liu SH, Henry MH, Nuccion SL. A prospective evaluation of a new physical examination in predicting glenoid labral tears. *Am J Sports Medicine* 1996; **24(6):** 721–725

20. Snyder SJ, Banas MP, Karzel RP. An analysis of 140 injuries to the superior glenoid labrum. *J Shoulder Elbow Surg.*1995; **4:** 243–248

21. Constant CR, Murley AHG. A clinical method of functional assessment of the shoulder. *Clin Orthop* 1987; **214:** 160–164

6

Examination of the Brachial Plexus Following Trauma

S Kay

Anatomy

The brachial plexus is most commonly formed by the coalescence of nerve fibres from the C5 C6 C7 C8 and T1 spinal nerves. It emerges from the interscalene space passing in the coronal plane laterally and caudally beneath the clavicle in that bone's central third and above the first rib. It emerges from beneath the clavicle to pass deep to the muscles attached to the coracoid process before finally entering the axilla and upper arm from behind the lateral border of pectoralis major. It has important relationships throughout this course, and these relationships bear upon the signs that may accompany damage to the plexus.

Anatomical relationships

The skeletal relationships are most easily understood. The spinal column lies medial to the plexus and may be caught up in the same zone of trauma. The clavicle and first rib may each be fractured, and damage to the first rib is associated with the dissipation of large amounts of kinetic energy. In exceptional circumstances fracture of the scapula and clavicle may indicate that the arm has suffered a near avulsion injury: a brachiothoracic dissociation, and that integrity of the skin envelope hides substantial deep trauma.

Two important neural associations with the brachial plexus are the sympathetic nerves and the phrenic nerve. The sympathetic rami for the arm and face emerge from the T1 root immediately after it exits the cervical foramen. Avulsion of this root therefore carries a high incidence of Horner's Syndrome (ptosis of the upper eyelid, meiosis of the pupil (smaller diameter), anhydrosis (loss of sweating on one half of the face: not easily demonstrated) and enophthalmos (not usually seen in the early stages). The phrenic nerve arises from the C5 root as it lies on the medial scalene muscle and receives its main contribution from C4. Phrenic nerve palsy is therefore most likely to indicate avulsion of the C5 root with or without avulsion of the C4 root. In the latter case other signs of cervical plexus palsy may include numbness over the lateral neck and ear, or rarely, trapezius palsy from involvement of the closely associated spinal accessory nerve.

The vascular relationships of the brachial plexus are most important, for not only do they provide evidence of collateral damage in cases of brachial plexus palsy, but that damage may itself be of great importance. As the T1 spinal nerve arches cephalad and lateral to join C8 at the first rib and so form the lower trunk, it also approaches the subclavian artery which crosses the first rib immediately anterior to the plexus and then lies intimately associated with it for the remainder of it's course. The artery is therefore susceptible to injury in the same manner as the T1 nerve root, and penetrating or avulsion injuries of the plexus are often associated with vascular damage. Arterial damage attracts greater attention than that to the subclavian vein.

Neural topography

The plexiform pattern of nerve coalescence and division is the result of the complex phylogenetic changes in the human limb as it evolved and assumed its current form. The pattern is variable and many find it difficult to recall. In fact it is in outline very simple. Three trunks bring nerve fibres to the plexus (the upper and lower are formed by the 2 most cephalad and the 2 most caudad roots) and each trunk divides into anterior and posterior divisions. These six divisions then regroup to form three cords named for their relationship to the axillary vessels, and then each cord contributes to the four major nerves that enter the upper arm.

The radial nerve is formed mainly from the posterior cord, whilst the medial cord forms the ulnar and part of the median nerve, the rest of the median coming from that part of the lateral cord that does not become the musculocutaneous nerve.

Some key nerves leave this plexus at important points and these are indicated in **Figure 1**.

Knowledge of this neural topography helps the examining surgeon to establish an anatomical map of the parts of the plexus not functioning, and so to localise the lesion. In practice this localisation is usually confined to estimating whether the injury is supraclavicular or infraclavicular, and how many roots are affected.

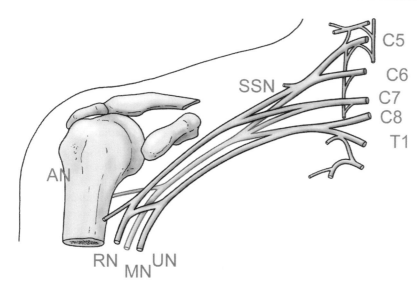

Figure 1 Brachial plexus with division into roots, trunks and cords together with branches. The roots C5 through T1 are shown. [SSN, suprascapular nerve; UN, Ulnar nerve; MN, median nerve; RN, Radial nerve; AN axillary nerve.]

Examination

The examination should be considered in three phases depending on how long has elapsed since the trauma.

1. Immediate Aftermath of Trauma

As with any trauma the simple life support principles of screening for major life threatening injury should be obeyed. In the case brachial plexus injury (BPI) the receiving surgeon should be especially alert to threats to the adjacent structures, i.e. the cervical spine, the great vessels and the thoracic cavity and contents. At this stage, the examination, having excluded life-threatening injury, should note the extent of the paralysis and sensory loss and chart this accurately where possible. Often pain and distress will make this examination incomplete, but any hard data should be recorded for future comparison. The examiner must be aware of the possibility of a Horner's syndrome in lower trunk injury, in which case the pupil inequality may be mistaken for a sign of cerebral damage. The vascular status of the limb should also be established and recorded, and evidence of subclavian artery rupture may include expanding supraclavicular haematoma.

Immediately post-trauma

Examination
Exclude life-threatening injury (standard ATLS primary survey)
Look for injury to adjacent structures
   Cervical spine
   Brain
   Subclavian vessels and mediastinal vessels
   Throracic cavity and contents
   Appendicular skeleton
Chart extent of sensory and motor loss as far as possible.
   Pinwheel, power tendon reflexes.
   Horner's syndrome
   Phrenic nerve
Examine the lower limb for long tract signs.

Investigations
CXR
   Fractures
   Widened mediastimum
   Phrenic nerve paralysis
Cervical spine X-ray
   Fracture or instability
Limb X-rays if insensate: especially wrist and forearm.
Angiography if vascular disturbance

Routine investigation at this early stage should include for all patients' cervical spine films and chest X-rays. In cases with extensive sensory loss in the arm, unappreciated fractures should be sought, especially of the wrist and forearm, where relatively subtle injuries can in the long term determine final outcome if undetected and untreated.

2. When Condition Stabilised

When appropriate care has been given to the urgent treatment of fractures and any visceral or vascular injuries, the patient may be assessed in more detail. This is the first opportunity to detect and record important data that will have bearing in the days to come when deciding whether clinical signs are evolving. The use of a standard brachial plexus chart for recording the findings is useful but not essential. A simple scheme is to record sensory findings on a sketch of the limb, and to record motor findings by muscle group or by movement.

General examination

Examine for signs of head injury, reiterate examination of cervical spine and look for a Horner's syndrome. Note coexisting injuries.

Where possible, the initial examination is facilitated if the patient is standing. The examiner should also stand and should begin by observation, inspecting the anterior and posterior aspects of the patient, noting posture, symmetry and signs of other injuries as well as tropic changes and evidence of surgical treatment. If the patient is unable to stand the reason should be determined, and in particular spinal causes should be excluded, bearing in mind that avulsion of the roots of the plexus may be associated with long tract signs.

Horner's syndrome should be sought. Horner's syndrome indicates an injury to the T1 root immediately after exiting from the foramen, and this is usually associated with avulsion of this root

A useful sign in this situation and in all peripheral nerve injuries is Tinel's phenomenon. The principle underlying this sign is that the injured axon and the

Table 1   The features of Horner's syndrome
Meiosis
Constricted pupil in the absence of sympathetic tone
Anhydrosis
Unilateral loss of sweating in the face
Ptosis
Drooping of the upper eyelid due to loss of sympathetic tone in Muller's muscle
Enophthalmos
Cause unknown

new growth cones of the regenerating nerve depolarise on mechanical stimulation. Percussion at the site of a significant nerve injury (*see* diagram) results in the patient perceiving tingling *distal* to the injury in the distribution of that nerve (whether motor or sensory). This is a reliable localising sign of nerve injury but it should be remembered that this sign may be present at the site of distal regeneration also. The Tinel's sign is not quantitative and the presence of a migrating Tinel's phenomenon indicates some fibres are regenerating and its position tells how advanced that process is, but does not indicate the eventual extent of recovery (**Figure 2**).

Sensory examination

The sensory examination for different modalities is important, but in the first instance the initial assessment is seeking areas of gross sensory loss and the most expedient way to undertake this is with a pinwheel (pain or nociception: **Figure 3**). This offers a measure of *threshold* assessment, and this may be supplemented by light touch using the examiners own fingertips (light touch). In each case the perception of each stimulus should be compared to the uninjured side (if such exists), and the patient asked to comment on difference and similarity. Such examination may sometimes be usefully supplemented by examining other sensory modalities if a neuropraxia or conduction block is suspected, for in these injuries some fibres are preferentially affected, leading to a predictable loss of one modality before another (**Figure 4**).

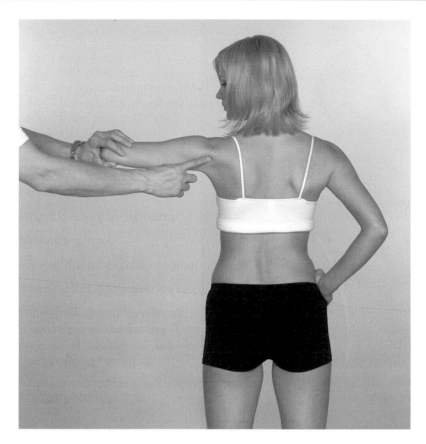

Figure 7 How to separate deltoid and supraspinatus function. Extension of the shoulder in this position tests the posterior fibres of the deltoid.

initiate abduction, whereas deltoid alone cannot. Conversely, supraspinatus can sustain abduction as can deltoid. In 90 degrees of abduction the most powerful extender of the glenohumeral joint is deltoid (posterior fibres). Weakness of supraspinatus may be distinguished from a rotator cuff tear with difficulty. External rotation is compromised and if no contraction of supraspinatus can be felt, imaging of the joint or direct inspection may be required.

Shoulder adduction is achieved mainly with two large muscles (pectoralis major and latissimus dorsi) that derive their innervation from several roots each, and so offers little localising information in terms of root involvement, but preservation of these muscles suggests involvement of the plexus distally, since the pectoral nerves emerge from the plexus early, and the thoracodorsal nerve emerges from the posterior trunk. A qualitative appreciation of latissimus dorsi function can be obtained by grasping the anterior free borders of both muscles and asking the patient to cough, exploiting the role of this muscle as an accessory muscle of respiration.

Scapular stability is provided by a large number of muscles, prime amongst which are the rhomboids, serratus anterior (again the long thoracic nerve derives innervation from several roots and so offers little localising information), and the trapezius (spinal accessory nerve: rarely injured). Paralysis of any of these three main muscles may result in an appearance of winging, which is not always due to long thoracic nerve palsy.

Elbow flexion is primarily a reflection of C6 with a little help from C5 and the three main flexors of the elbow offer specific information about the cords and nerves. *Biceps brachii* is innervated by the musculocutaneous nerve (lateral cord) as is the *brachialis* (predominantly musculocutaneous but some radial nerve laterally) whilst the *brachioradialis* is innervated by the radial nerve (posterior cord). Elbow flexion should initially be tested without the effects gravity (**Figure 8**). Further assessment should record range of elbow flexion and weight lifted or resistance.

Elbow extension is predominantly C7 innervated triceps, from the radial nerve (posterior cord) and should be tested in a similar fashion to biceps.

Wrist extension is also predominantly C7 with some input from C8 and is via the radial nerve (posterior cord).

Finger and thumb extension at the metacarpophalangeal joints is predominantly C7, 8. Extension at

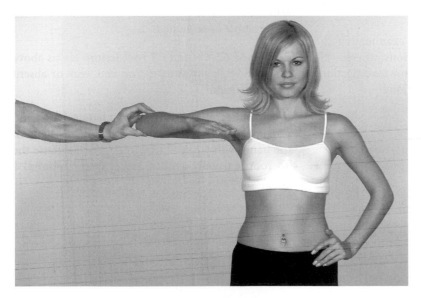

Figure 8 How to test elbow flexion without the effects of gravity.

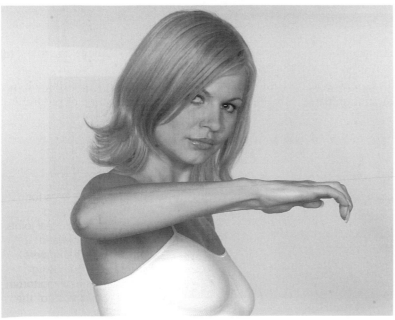

Figure 9 Extension of metacarpo-phalangeal joints assessing extrinsic extensors.

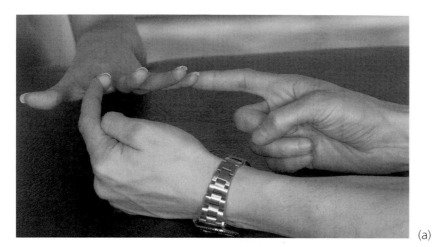

(a)

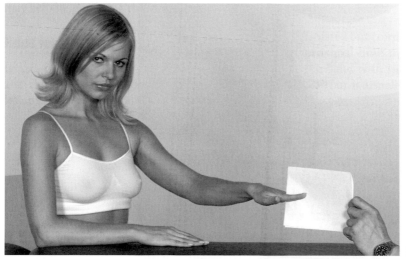

(b)

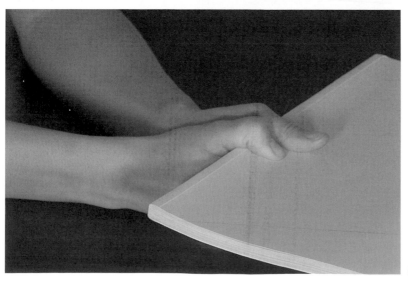

(c)

Figure 11, a, b, c Tests for finger abduction and adduction. Froment's test (c) demonstrates how weak intrinsics lead to the recruitment of the long flexor of the thumb.

Investigations

Imaging

Radiographs may have already given some information about adjacent skeletal injuries that provide clues to the extent of injury. Myelography may be employed and show myeloceles (presumptive evidence of intradural injury, which may or may not be complete) or may define the intradural rootlets or their absence. Combined with a CT scan the sensitivity of this investigation is increased, but false positives and negatives can occur in up to 5% of cases. More recently MRI studies have yielded similar results in some units.

Electrical studies

Electrophysiology adds little to the clinical findings in the co-operative awake patient at this stage unless it is necessary to exclude the possibility of a conduction block or neuropraxia. In the unconscious poly trauma patient such studies may be useful.

Treatment

The key question at this stage and assuming other injuries permit is whether or not surgery is immediately indicated. Opinions vary on the precise indications but as a general rule some observations may be made. Firstly the primary intent of surgery is diagnosis. No clinical inference or imaging study will substitute for a direct experienced examination of the plexus from foramina to axilla. This is however a considerable undertaking, and should be done only in the expectation of finding pathology that can then be immediately treated. Thus the examination aims to predict that pathology and to shape a plan for treatment and fall back options that can be discussed prior to surgery and completed at surgery. The surgeon must identify those cases likely to have suffered nerve rupture or avulsion. Some findings argue strongly for such findings, namely a history of high-energy trauma, more than one root or nerve involved completely, and clinical or imaging signs of avulsion.

3. The Late Stage

Faced with a patient many months after injury the surgeon will have to answer different questions. The results of exploration and repair are poorer after 6 months and in general not worthwhile for restoration of motor function in adults after 1 year, although some improvement in sensibility may occur. At this stage the surgeon will be examining the patient with a view to secondary reconstruction, and the options here are numerous. In general they consist of osteotomy, arthrodeses and tendon transfers, and in some cases nerve transfers to power free functioning muscle transfers. For these reasons the surgeon will need to evaluate the degree of recovery and determine whether further recovery is taking place. He or she will be interested in the function of the hand, and it's supporting structures and in determining whether the injury is primarily upper root or lower root. In upper root palsy the hand may function very well but the patient may lack the vital positioning qualities of a stable shoulder, together with external rotation and elbow flexion. In the converse situation, absent lower root function may leave good shoulder or elbow function with little hand use, raising doubts about the value of complex proximal reconstruction.

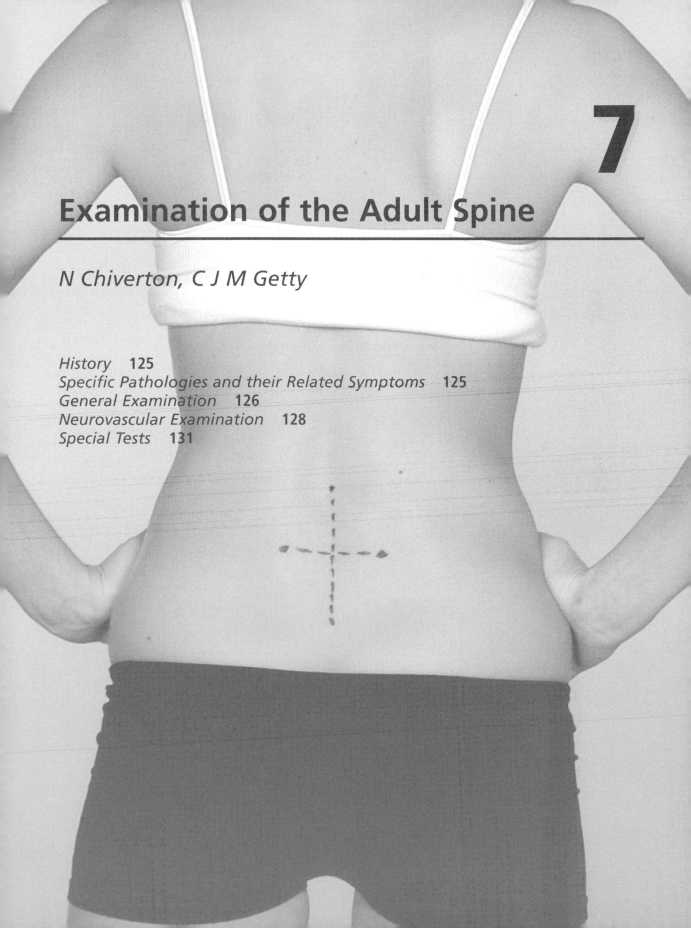

7

Examination of the Adult Spine

N Chiverton, C J M Getty

History

General history

The majority of adult patients with problems of spinal origin present with complaints of pain in the back and/or legs, with a resultant loss of function.

It is, therefore, as important to understand and record the impact of the perceived pain on the daily work and recreational activities of the patient as it is to enquire about the nature of the pain itself.

One should begin with the patient's occupation, social circumstances (e.g. young children at home, carer for elderly relative, living alone) and sporting activities. One can then proceed to enquire about the limitations on all of these aspects of daily living with particular reference to days taken off work, time periods of relative immobility and problems coping with household duties. Specific disability scoring systems[1, 2] can be used if wished. The patient's age should always be used to help steer your thoughts towards a likely diagnosis. Never accept a diagnosis of mechanical back pain in patients outside an age range of 20–55 years without thorough investigation, particularly in the presence of non-mechanical or other atypical symptoms.

With regard to the pain, one should record its site, radiation, any precipitating or relieving factors (e.g. posture, cough/sneeze, physical activity), causation, duration and any pain free intervals.

It is essential to enquire directly about any bowel or bladder dysfunction.

Additionally, it is important to take note of whether the patient considers his/her back problem to be work related and whether or not there are any legal proceedings pending.

One must take care, however, not to let these facts influence one's early judgments, although they may prove pertinent after examination and appropriate investigations have not revealed an abnormality consistent with the reported symptoms.

The requirements for analgesics and their effectiveness are a useful guide for the clinician as to the degree of pain experienced by the patient. Also ask about any previous treatments received such as physiotherapy or chiropractic therapy.

The history taking should, as always, conclude with a systems review, past medical history, family history, other medications, and allergies. With regard to back pain, heredity is also important.

Specific Pathologies and their Related Symptoms

Degenerative disease of the cervical spine

Pain in the neck may be a symptom of cervical spondylosis. Other causes of referred pain to the neck such as shoulder girdle pathology and cervical soft tissue tumours should be considered. Neck stiffness is often reported.

In severe cases of spondylosis patients can present with symptoms of compressive cervical myelopathy, cervical radiculopathy, or a mixture of both.

Unsteadiness of gait, limb weakness and sensory disturbance in the upper or lower limbs, and urinary dysfunction are the cardinal symptoms of a cervical myelopathy. Patients will commonly report an episodic rather than a gradual deterioration. A thorough history will be required if metabolic, rheumatological, and primary neural degenerative disorders are not to be overlooked as potential causes of these symptoms.

Acute cervical disc protrusion can cause myelopathic symptoms, but classically will present with neck and arm pain (brachalgia), the latter resulting from nerve root compression and being the most troublesome to the patient. It is usually described as a burning/toothache type pain. Sensory disturbance is frequently associated. The site of the upper limb pain varies according to the disc level involved, most common are the C5/6 and C6/7 disc levels affecting the C6 and C7 nerve roots respectively. This gives rise to pain and parasthesiae along the radial aspect of the forearm and into the radial digits. A differential diagnosis based on these symptoms will include peripheral nerve entrapment syndromes, thoracic outlet syndrome, tumours abutting the brachial plexus, idiopathic brachial neuritis and spinal tumours.

A painless but progressive flexion deformity of the cervical spine progressing from a limitation of the forward field of view to difficulty with jaw opening characterises the cervical spinal manifestations of ankylosing spondylitis.

Degenerative disease of the lumbar spine

A history of low back pain proportional to activity level with periods of exacerbation lasting 2–6 weeks and with radiation into the gluteal and thigh regions only is indicative of so called 'discogenic pain' from degenerative lower lumbar motion segments. Any associated pain or sensory disturbance in the lower leg or foot suggests the co-existence of a compressive radiculopathy. If the cause of this is an acute intervertebral disc protrusion the leg pain tends to be severe, unilateral and exacerbated by posture.

The most likely disc level involved can usually be appreciated by ascertaining where the patient reports the symptoms of leg pain, tingling or numbness.

Any reported bowel or bladder disturbance necessitates further investigation, as does reduced perineal sensation.

Neurogenic bladder dysfunction presents as painless overflow incontinence. Symptoms of prostatic hypertrophy in men and stress or urge incontinence in women are not consistent with a cauda equina syndrome and careful differentiation is essential before urgent investigations are requested unnecessarily.

Back pain with leg pain after a certain period of time walking or standing is suggestive of spinal claudication. Leg symptoms are commonly bilateral and the reported distribution less specific than with an isolated nerve root compression. Patients with spinal claudication will frequently report improvement in symptoms when walking by leaning on a walking stick, shopping trolley or when walking uphill as these flexed postures increase spinal canal diameter. Complete relief is achieved by sitting for several

minutes. In the more severe cases rest and night symptoms are present ('restless legs') and neurogenic bladder dysfunction can occur. The differential diagnosis of vascular claudication can be difficult to exclude on history alone but is usually relieved by standing still as well as sitting and symptoms resolve more rapidly.

Other differential diagnoses include diabetic or alcoholic peripheral neuropathy, and spinal tumours.

A combination of radicular and stenotic symptoms as outlined above should raise the possibility of degenerative lumbar spondylolisthesis in which both spinal canal compromise and nerve root entrapment result from the forward slip of one complete vertebra on another.

Degenerative disease of the thoracic spine

Pathology involving the thoracic spine is rare with, for instance, only 0.5% of all disc protrusions occurring in this region. However, they should be considered in anyone complaining of inter-scapular back pain. The pain has the same nature and precipitating factors as are found in equivalent conditions of the lumbar spine. Radicular symptoms are felt around the chest wall in the distribution of corresponding intercostal nerve. Myelopathy may affect bladder and bowel function as well as all lower limb muscle groups.

Differential diagnoses include herpes zoster, mediastinal or abdominal pathology and, as always, spinal tumours.

General Examination

Inspection

Examination of any localised spinal disorder requires inspection of the entire spine. All patients must undress to their underwear for this to be possible.

The usual format for inspection should be followed, firstly noting any obvious swellings or surgical scars.

The erect spinal profile must be assessed for any deformity in the coronal or sagittal plane. Scoliosis will be due to either a previous developmental deformity or to degenerative disease of later onset, or both. A 'forward bend test' may reveal the presence of a rib hump seen commonly in the former, but uncommonly in the latter. Kyphosis in the region of the cervicothoracic junction is typically seen with ankylosing spondylitis, whereas in the thoracic region it is likely to represent either previous Scheuermann's disease or multiple osteoporotic wedge fractures. Loss of lordosis in the lumbar spine is commonly seen in association with protective paravertebral muscle spasm secondary to underlying degenerative disease. Hyperlordosis should raise the suspicion of spondylolisthesis. Prominent buttocks, shortened trunk, and flexed hips and knees may be seen with severe slips. A compensatory lumbar hyperlordosis will be found below a primary thoracic kyphotic deformity.

One should follow this assessment with a check for shoulder asymmetry and pelvic tilt. A plumbline can be used to quantify any coronal imbalance if wished.

Finally, the patient must be observed walking. An antalgic gait is often noted in the presence of lumbar radiculopathy secondary to disc prolapse. A broad based unsteady gait can be seen in advanced cervical myelopathy.

Palpation

Palpation along the line of the spine over the paravertebral muscles on both sides is very non-specific, but helps to localise the level of the spine involved. Often a region of tenderness on deep palpation is found. Very localised points of tenderness on deep muscle palpation are suggestive of fibromyalgia. Occasionally one may encounter marked superficial tenderness, or a non-anatomic distribution of tenderness which may be non-organic in nature[3], but one must keep an open mind at this stage as the former sign may be elicited in destructive or infective lesions of the spine.

Palpation should be completed with an abdominal examination to identify any masses, especially a distended neurogenic bladder and the obligatory PR examination of sensation, anal tone and prostate.

Movement

All spinal movements are best assessed actively by instructing the patient on the movements required, but some passive movements are useful.

For the cervical spine movements of flexion, extension, rotation, and lateral flexion should be assessed. Flexion and extension are mostly affected by spondylosis. A tendency to hold the head on one side with radicular arm pain when the neck is gently passively laterally flexed to the other side suggests a cervical disc prolapse (on the contralateral side to the active lateral flexion). Normally, only 40% of rotational movement occurs in the subaxial spine so this movement is well preserved in most degenerative disorders.

Facet joint orientation and the splinting effect of the thoracic cage allow for essentially only rotational movement in the thoracic spine. Assessment of this movement is, however, of little diagnostic significance. Conversely, because of the orientation of the facet joints in the lumbar spine little rotation is possible and flexion/extension movements are examined.

Measurement of forward bending is performed by asking the patient to try and touch their toes. Note and record to what extent they can achieve this (e.g. fingers to knees, mid shin, toes). One should ensure by inspection that the movement is achieved by flexion of the lumbar spine and not the hips only.

Schober's Test[4] can be used to provide a more quantitative evaluation of lumbar spine flexion. Mark a first horizontal line at the level of PSIS's and a second at a distance of 10cm. above this. On forward flexion this distance should increase by at least 5cm. (**Figure 1a**). A modification of this test[5] uses a distal fixed point 5 cm below the PSIS line and the same point above (**Figure 1b**). Limitation of flexion is due to pain protection or ankylosing spondylitis.

When testing extension stand behind the patient supporting and reassuring them. The limitation here can be more marked than limitation of flexion in degenerative disease and is said to indicate facet joint arthrosis.

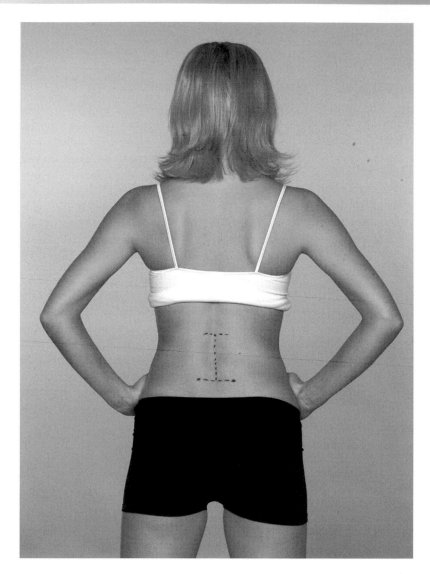

Figure 1a A 10 cm line extending from the posterior superior iliac spines cephalad as described in Schober's Test. With flexion this should increase at least 5 cm in length.

Essential adjuncts to examination of the cervical and lumbar spine are screening movements of the shoulder and hip joints respectively to exclude them as a cause of the pain in these regions.

Neurovascular Examination

A thorough, orderly examination of sensation, tone, power, and reflexes must be performed on the all four limbs for problems with the cervical spine and

on the lower limbs for thoracolumbar disease. A summary of muscle innervation and reflex values (**Tables 1a** and **1b**) and dermatomal distributions (**Figure 2**) are given, but the reader is directed to the MRC booklet on neurological testing[6] for more detailed descriptions. See 'special tests' below for other specific tests.

All peripheral pulses need to be checked as vascular claudication in the upper or lower limbs can mimic symptoms of radiculopathy or canal stenosis.

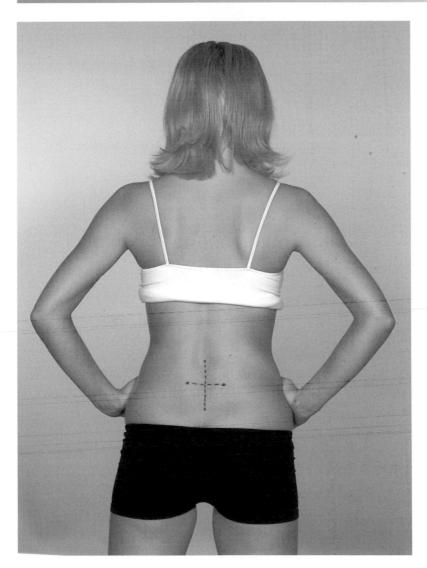

Figure 1b A modification of Schober's Test – the line running from 5 cm below the posterior superior iliac spines to 5 cm above the posterior superior iliac spines.

Table 1a The muscle innervation and reflex values of the upper limb muscles

Action	Principle Muscles	Major Root Values
Shoulder abduction	Supraspinatus / deltoid	C5
Elbow flexion	Brachialis / Biceps brachii	C5, C6
Wrist extension	Extensor carpi radialis / ulnaris	C6, C7
Elbow extension	Triceps	C6, C7, C8
Finger extension	Extensor digitorum / pollicis / indicis	C7, C8
Finger flexion	Flexor pollicis / digitorum communis	C8
Finger abduction	Dorsal interossei	C8, T1
Finger adduction	Palmar interossei	C8, T1

Table 1b The muscle innervation and reflex values of the lower limb muscles

Action	Principle Muscles	Major Root Values
Hip flexion	Iliopsoas	L1, L2
Hip adduction	Adductor longus / magnus	L2, L3
Knee extension	Quadriceps femoris	L3, L4
Foot dorsiflexion	Tibialis anterior	L4
Toe extension	Extensor digitorum / hallucis	L5
Hip abduction	Gluteus medius / minimis	L4, L5
Hip extension	Gluteus maximus	L5, S1
Knee flexion	Hamstrings	S1
Foot plantar flexion	Gastrocnemius and soleus	S1, S2
Toe flexion	Flexor digitorum / hallucis longus	S1, S2

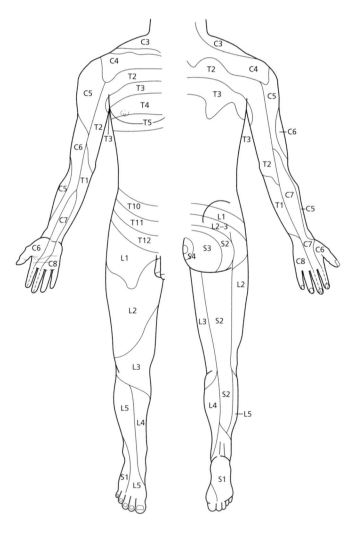

Ventral   Dorsal   **Figure 2** Dermatomal distributions.

Special Tests

Cervical spine

Symptoms of cervical radiculopathy can be exacerbated by Spurling's manoeuvre,[7] which narrows the involved neuroforamen. The neck is gently hyperextended, then laterally flexed and rotated to the side of the suspected lesion. Significant relief of symptoms with subsequent abduction of the ipsilateral shoulder (Shoulder Abduction Relief Test) lends further support to the diagnosis of intervertebral disc herniation. A positive Tinel's sign can sometimes be elicited over the exiting nerve root.

If there is suspicion of thoracic outlet syndrome such as pain and parasthesiae in the arm with overhead activity, turning the head to one side or deep inspiration (especially with C8 and T1 symptoms) provocative tests for obliteration of the radial pulse or reproduction of symptoms can be performed[8]. In Adson's manoeuvre, the head is extended and rotated to the affected side. The arm is abducted 15° and the radial pulse felt. Obliteration of the pulse with deep inspiration or loss of the pulse whilst maintaining the same position whilst breathing normally is suggestive of thoracic outlet syndrome.[9] Roos[10] described abducting the shoulders and flexing the elbows to 90°. In this position the shoulders are braced backwards and the patient is asked to rapidly flex and extend the fingers. Reproduction of the symptoms is thought to be indicative of thoracic outlet syndrome.

Peripheral nerve entrapments must also be excluded by appropriate tests discussed in the relevant chapter when numbness, paraesthesia, and weakness are reported in the upper limb. Remember also that radiculopathy and peripheral nerve entrapments may co-exist and in these cases EMGs and nerve conduction studies will be required to elucidate the major contributor to the symptoms.

Flexion of the neck which precipitates lightning pains or parasthaesia in the lower limbs represents L'hermitte's sign and is characteristic of cervical spinal myelopathy. Other important long tract signs in the assessment of this condition are:

- The plantar responses – when performing this test use a gentle stroke with your thumb nail.

The use of the pointed end of a reflex hammer or objects such as a car key is to be avoided.

- Clonus at the ankle or knee – more than three beats is an abnormal finding.
- Hoffman's sign - flexion of the thumb and index finger following a flick to the pulp of the index finger
- Inverted radial reflex – finger flexion seen with the brachioradialis tendon reflex

Lumbar spine

Signs of lumbar nerve root irritation, most commonly due to an intervertebral disc protrusion, may be observed when performing a series of tests. These tests rely on reproducing / exacerbating pain in the affected leg and should therefore be performed at the conclusion of the examination and in the order described.

With the patient lying supine slowly raise the affected leg; supporting it with the palm of the hand under the heel, rather than grasping the ankle. Ensure there is no knee flexion. When the patient complains of pain (usually between 30–60° of elevation) stop and ask whether the pain is being experienced in the back or down the leg (**Figure 3a**). This is the straight leg raise test. If the leg is then lowered a little to relieve the discomfort and the foot passively dorsiflexed the pain may be reproduced again (**Figure 3b**). This is Lasègue's sign.[11]

Next, with the knee and hip flexed to 45°, the 'bowstring test' can be carried out by pressing behind the knee over the popliteal nerve with one's thumb. If leg pain is reproduced this indicates sciatic nerve tension (**Figure 3c**). With true sciatic irritation, pressure over the medial or lateral hamstring tendons should not give a positive result.

Finally, with both legs again now flat on the couch and one hand placed gently on the knees to keep them in extension the patient is asked to sit forward. In the presence of nerve root tension the patient will not be able to sit upright with the knees fully extended (**Figure 3d**).

The 'Flip Test' is a variation of the last manoeuvre. Sit the patient upright with their knees flexed over

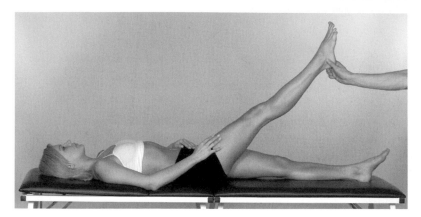

Figure 3a The straight leg raise. The palm is placed under the heel with the leg extended. Only a reproduction of pain down the leg with elevation is regarded as positive not an exacerbation of back pain.

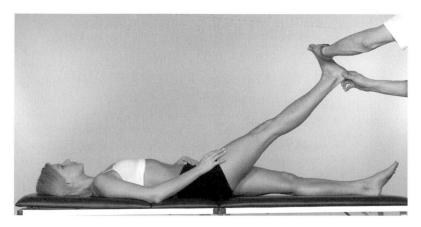

Figure 3b Passive dorsiflexion of the foot increases root tension and reinforces a positive straight leg raise.

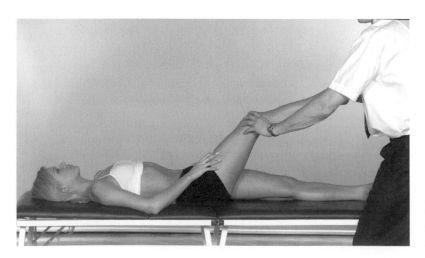

Figure 3c The hip and knee flexed 45° with pressure in the popliteal fossa again serving to increase root tension.

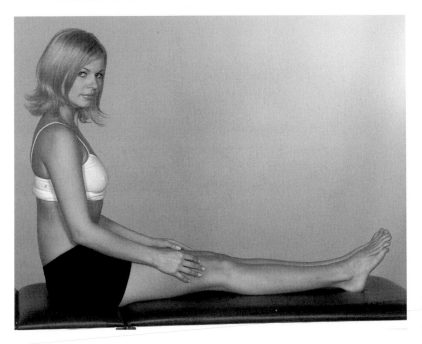

Figure 3d The patient sitting upright on the examination couch with the legs extended. This is equivalent to a 90° straight leg raise.

the edge of the couch, actively extend the knees in turn. This should produce the same response as the SLR test in the genuine patient.

A straight leg raise test performed on the unaffected leg which gives rise to pain in the affected leg, the 'crossover sign' has been reported to indicate that the disc protrusion lies in the axilla of the nerve root rather than in the more common lateral position, but this correlation is not reliable.

Finally, with the patient now lying in the prone position the Femoral Stretch Test can be performed. With the knee passively flexed to 90° and a hand gently keeping the pelvis against the couch lift the foot upwards and note the distribution of any pain provoked by this manoeuvre.

References

1. Fairbank CJT, Davies JB, Couper J, O'Brien JP. The Oswestry low back pain disability questionnaire. *Physiotherapy* 1980; **66:** 271–273

2. Ware JE Jnr., Snow KK, Kosinski M, Gandek B. SF-36 Health Survey; Manual and Interpretation Guide. Boston. The Health Institute, 1993

3. Waddell G, McCulloch JA, Kummel E, Venner RM. Nonorganic physical signs in low-back pain. *Spine* 1980; **5(2):** 117–12

4. Schober P. (Lendenwirbelsaule und Kreuzschmerzen). *Munch Med Wschr* 1937; **84:** 336

5. Macrea IF, Wright V. Measurement of back movement. *Ann Rheum Dis* 1969; **28:** 584–593

6. Medical Research Council. Aids to the examination of the peripheral nervous system. HMSO 1976

7. Spurling RG. *Lesions of the Cervical Intevertebral Disc.* Springfield IL: Thomas, 1956

8. Oates SD, Daley RA. Thoracic outlet syndrome. *Hand Clin* 1996; **12(4):** 705–18

9. Adson AW,Coffey JR. Cervical rib: a method of anterior approach for relief of symptoms by division of the scalenus anticus. *Ann Surg* 1927; **85:** 839–55

10. Roos D. Transaxillary approach for first rib resection to relieve thoracic outlet syndrome. *Ann Surg* 1966; **163:** 354–8

11. Lasègue C. Considerations sur la sciatique. *Arch Gen Med* 1864; **2:** 558

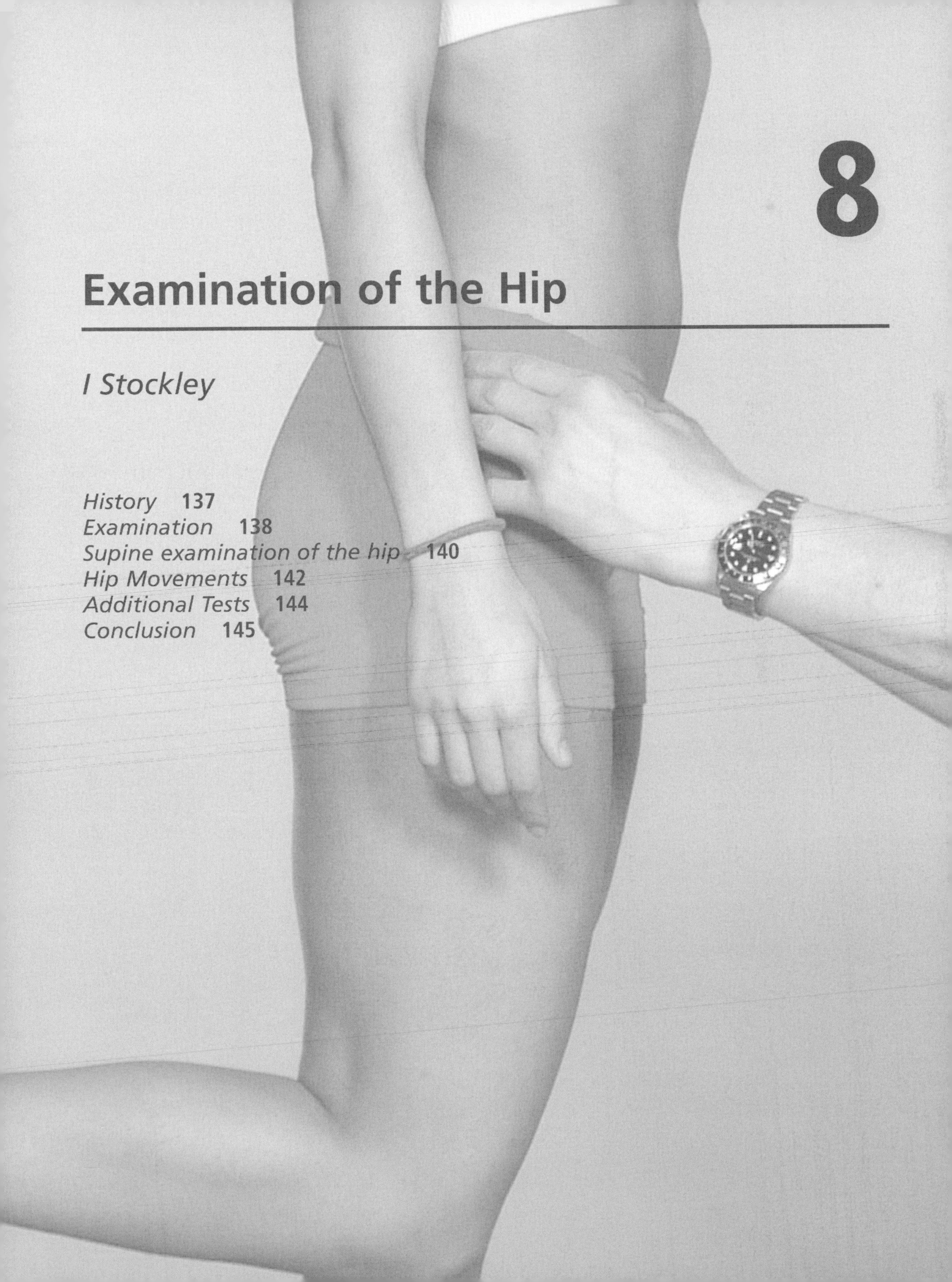

Examination of the Hip

I Stockley

8

History

A detailed clinical history and complete physical examination are mandatory in the assessment of the patient with a painful hip. Often a tentative diagnosis can be made on the history alone. Examination and subsequent investigations allow for confirmation or modification of the presumptive diagnosis.

Presenting complaints in hip pathology may include pain, limp and stiffness. Patients may not complain of stiffness per se but of the disability produced by it (e.g. the inability to put socks on). In trying to evaluate a patient's symptomatology it is important to know what effect if any the symptoms have on the patients' ability to undertake activities of everyday living.

It is important to ask patients whether they have had any previous problems with their hips. Childhood conditions affecting the hip may cause symptoms in early adult life because of the development of secondary degenerative changes. In addition, a history of previous surgery is very important when contemplating further surgical procedures as consideration needs to be given to previous scars, the surgical approach, skeletal deformity and in addition the increased risk of sepsis with arthroplasty surgery.

Several validated hip assessment scores are now available which allow for a more objective assessment of hip function. The Harris hip score is scored by the examiner and emphasizes range of motion, pain and function. The Oxford hip score and the WOMAC Osteoarthritis Index are scored by the patient and so remove any potential clinician bias. These scores if readministered after treatment are useful in objectively quantifying both how patients perceive the results of that treatment modality and whether it led to improved well-being and functional ability.

The patient's individual occupational and recreational demands need to be known when discussing management options. What is appropriate for one patient, may not be so for another, despite initial similarities.

Pain

Pain in the groin or thigh region is most likely a result of hip disease and is believed to arise from the joint capsule and synovial lining. Radiation to the anterior, medial or lateral thigh is common as is pain referred to the knee. Obviously, patients may have symptoms related to the knees as a direct consequence of knee pathology but referred pain from above always needs to be considered. "Hip pain" localised to the gluteal region is often referred pain from lumbosacral pathology and there may be associated radicular symptoms and signs. Differentiation between hip and back pain can usually be made on the basis of history, clinical examination and X-rays, but if in doubt an injection of local anaesthetic into the hip joint can be very useful.

Pain as a consequence of arthritis is usually exacerbated by exercise and relieved by rest. However, as the pathology progresses, pain at rest becomes a feature.

The differential diagnosis of a patient presenting with hip pain should always include infection. Pyogenic infection of the hip presents as pain localised to the groin or inner thigh. Pain secondary to infection is constant and unrelenting in character. The patient will experience pain with weight bearing but also have pain at rest. When pain is caused by haematogenous spread, the onset of pain is often acute and caused by distention of the joint capsule and secondary muscle spasm. A more insidious onset is the norm when the infection is by direct extension, as there is no dramatic increase in intra articular pressure.

Stiffness and limp

Patients do not often complain of stiffness but complain of the difficulties they have undertaking activities of everyday living as a consequence of the stiffness i.e. going up stairs, cutting toe nails and putting socks on etc. The term stiffness usually includes some loss of range of motion, it is a sensation experienced by the patient.

Limping can be due to a variety of reasons including; pain, limb length inequality, muscle weakness, and bone and joint deformity. If the hip is very stiff then patients often complain of a limp and not necessarily pain.

Snapping and clicky hips

Snapping and clicky hips tend to occur in adolescents and young adults. The patients often produce the symptoms and demonstrate the physical signs on demand and so tend to become habitual in nature. Intra-articular and extra-articular pathologies have been described. Although often there is no obvious abnormality detected either clinically or by investigation. Pain can be associated with the mechanical symptoms and radiates to the groin or laterally towards the greater trochanter area.

Examination

General

Examination starts as soon as the patient walks into the room. Are they using a cane or crutches? Is there a limp? Are they in pain? Often there are many clues, which can be explored later during the formal examination.

Inspection

With the patient standing barefoot and dressed down to underwear, muscle wasting and scars can be seen and posture is noted for the presence of contractures, spinal deformity and the ability to stand with feet, flat on the ground. A leg length discrepancy may now be seen and if present, could be assessed at this stage by asking the patient to stand on blocks of wood of varying height. The patient is asked "Do you feel level now?" and the blocks are changed as necessary until the patient feels level. This is probably a better assessment of leg length inequality than using a tape measure as the patient is actively involved in this assessment and it is how he or she feels when standing which is important rather than a measurement on a tape measure. Looking and palpating the iliac crests gives an assessment of pelvic obliquity, which will be corrected if the obliquity is due to leg length inequality. However, fixed obliquity due to lumbosacral disease cannot be compensated for in this manner.

The Trendelenburg test can now be performed to assess abductor function. Trendelenburg in 1895 described observations on the gait of congenital dislocated hip patients. He described how the upper body swings to the side of weight-bearing in a child with CDH. Later he went on to describe the pelvic inclination on single leg weight-bearing, which became known as the Trendelenburg test. This was originally described with the examiner standing behind the patient so that the dimples overlying the posterior superior iliac spines could be seen to move up and down when the test was being performed.

It is my experience, however that unless somebody is actually facing the patient, he or she is reluctant to stand on one leg particularly if the hip is painful. When performing the test, the patient is asked to stand on one leg with the hip and knee on the unsupported side flexed to 90° if possible (**Figure 1**). The test is negative i.e. the abductor mechanism is normal when the pelvis remains level. A positive result indicates abductor dysfunction and the pelvis on the unsupported side will descend. A patient standing on his right leg would be Trendelenburg positive for the right, if the left side dipped. A Trendelenburg can be positive for two main reasons, neurological or mechanical. Neurological causes can be due to generalised motor weakness as seen with myelomeningocele and spinal cord lesions or more specific problems e.g. superior gluteal nerve dysfunction. The mechanical group includes conditions that affect the abductor muscle lever arm (e.g. congenital dislocation of the hip, coxa vara and fractures). These conditions shorten the length of the muscle from its origin to its insertion and significantly weaken its strength.

It is important to be aware that patients who have a weakened abductor mechanism may not descend on one side when performing the Trendelenburg test, as they can compensate by leaning over the affected hip to shift the body's center of gravity in that direction. This is called a Trendelenburg lurch. However, patients with advanced arthritis of the hip may lurch towards the ipsilateral stance limb simply because the arthritis prevents the pelvic tilt and to maintain balance, the patient leans over.

The delayed Trendelenburg test is really non-specific. Any painful hip condition will be positive after the patient has been performing the test for 30 seconds to a minute. I personally question its value.

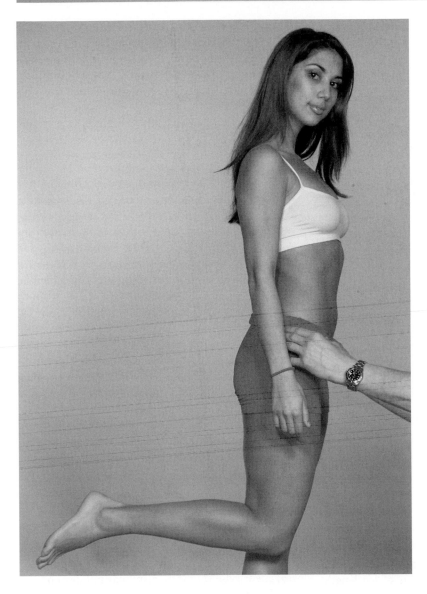

Figure 1 Trendelenberg Test –
the Surgeon faces the patients
and asks them to stand on one
leg. The hip and knee are flexed
to 90° on the unsupported side.
The pelvis should remain level or
rise. A positive result is when
the pelvis dips on the
unsupported side.

Gait

Abnormal pathology in the lower limb is often demonstrated by changes in the gait pattern whether it is a compensatory adaptation to pain, loss of motion or weakness.

Common gait patterns include:

- *Antalgic gait*: Pain in the hip on weight-bearing can be diminished by reducing the time spent on the affected leg (stance phase) and by leaning the trunk over to the symptomatic side when in stance phase. It also involves an excessive drop in the center of gravity as a means of reducing peak loading on weight-bearing. This produces an uneven stance period, which is the characteristic feature of an antalgic gait.

- *Short leg gait*: This involves excessive shift of the center of gravity toward the short side with a drop of the center of gravity. It differs from the antalgic gait in that the stance period is equal.

■ *Trendelenburg gait*: This is indicated by a drop of the pelvis on the opposite side to the stance limb. However, in order to maintain center of gravity above the stance limb it is not unusual for the trunk to lurch towards the ipsilateral stance limb.

■ *Gluteus maximus gait*: Hip extensor weakness (gluteus maximus) necessitates a forward thrust of the pelvis and backward thrust of the trunk. This position places the center of gravity posterior to the hip, tenses the iliofemoral ligament and stabilises the situation.

Supine examination of the hip

Palpation

The hip joint is too deep to assess for the presence of an effusion or synovial thickening. Bony landmarks can be palpated and include the anterior superior iliac spine and the greater trochanter.

As a preliminary step it is important to set the pelvis square. Determine from the position of the anterior superior iliac spines whether or not the pelvis is lying square with the limbs. If it is not, an attempt is made to set it square. If the pelvis cannot be squared up then there is a fixed adduction or abduction deformity at one or both hips. This should be noted.

Measurements of leg length

It is important to know whether any leg length inequality present is real or apparent. Although it is always necessary to measure for true discrepancy it is not so for apparent, unless there is fixed pelvic obliquity. Ideally it would be best to measure from the center of the femoral head, the normal axis of hip movement but as there is no surface landmark the nearest fixed point, the anterior superior iliac spine is chosen. Distally, measurements are taken to the medial malleolus. If there is a fixed deformity, the good leg must be placed in a comparably deformed position relative to the pelvis before measurements are taken (**Figure 2**). If not, measurements will be inaccurate as the angle between the leg and pelvis will be different on the two sides. Apparent shortening is measured from any midline point in the body e.g. umbilicus, xiphisternum. Adduction makes the limb appear shorter – each 10° of fixed adduction adds a further 3 cm of apparent

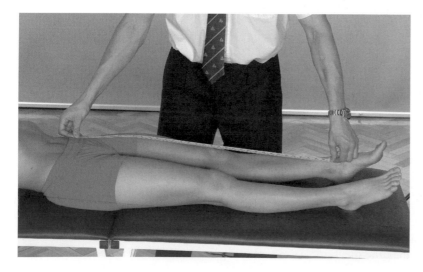

Figure 2 Real leg length measurements. The unaffected side is placed in the same position as the affected.

shortening to any real shortening which the disorder may have caused.

Is the shortening above or below the knee? If both knees are flexed while the heels remain on the couch, it can be seen whether shortening is in the femur or tibia (**Figure 3**). Having determined that the limb length inequality is in the femur, is it above the trochanter (suggesting a problem in or near the hip joint) or below the trochanter? X-rays would obviously tell the answer but there are clinical measurements that can be taken. However, in every day clinical practice they are not often used. The tests described for shortening above the greater trochanter include Bryant's triangle, Nelaton's line and Schoemaker's line.

Bryant's triangle

With the patient lying supine, a perpendicular is dropped from the anterior superior spine of the

ilium and meets a second line projected upwards from the tip of the greater trochanter. The length of this second line is compared between the two sides. Relative shortening on one side indicates that the femur is displaced upwards as a consequence of a problem in or near the hip joint. If the pathology is bilateral, Bryant's triangle is not helpful (**Figure 4**).

Nelaton's line

The patient lies with the affected side uppermost. A tape measure or string is stretched from the ischial tuberosity to the anterior iliac spine. Normally the greater trochanter lies on or below the line and so if the trochanter lies above the line, the femur has been displaced proximally (**Figure 5**).

Schoemaker's line

A line is projected on each side of the body from the greater trochanter through and beyond the anterior

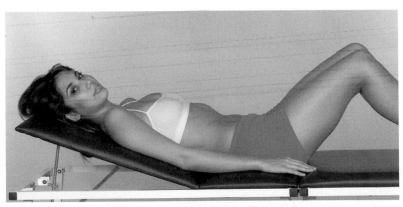

(a)

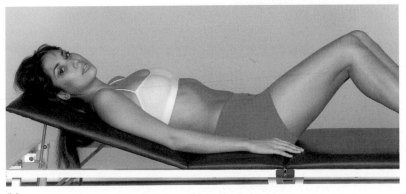

(b)

Figure 3 Placing both heels together on the examination couch allows the examiner to determine whether a leg length discrepancy is above or below the knee.
(a) Tibial shortening causes the affected knee to lie lower than the unaffected side.
(b) Femoral shortening causes the knee to adopt a more proximal position.

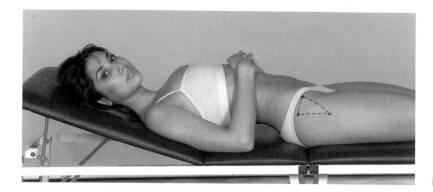

Figure 4 Bryant's Triangle.

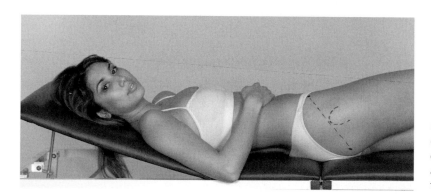

Figure 5 Nelaton's line. The greater trochanter should lie on or below a line connecting the anterior superior iliac spine and the ischial tuberosity.

superior iliac spine. Normally the two lines meet in the midline above the umbilicus. If there is a proximal femoral problem the lines will meet away from the midline on the opposite side. If the problem is bilateral the lines will meet at or near the midline but below the umbilicus.

Hip Movements

Active and passive movements of the hips should be recorded. Measurements should include flexion and extension, abduction and adduction, internal and external rotation both in flexion and extension. There is considerable variation in the "normal" range of motion among individuals. The patient with hip pathology may well have significant reduction in movement secondary to pain and degenerative changes. The accurate determination of hip movements needs care as restriction of hip movement is easily masked by movement of the pelvis. It is therefore essential to place one hand on the pelvis while the other supports and moves the leg.

Flexion

Hip flexion is normally tested in the supine position with the knee flexed to prevent hamstring tightness restricting movement. In the normal hip, flexion is limited by the soft tissues of the thigh and abdomen. Rotation of the pelvis increasing the range of flexion is best detected by grasping the crest of the ilium. Normal flexion is recorded from 0° to between 100 and 135°.

The primary flexor of the hip is the iliopsoas muscle. Muscle power is assessed by having the patient sitting on the edge of the examination couch with the legs dangling down. The patient is then asked to raise the thigh from the table. The examiner places his hands on the distal thigh and assesses muscle power.

Contracture of the joint capsule will cause deformity. Fixed flexion, fixed adduction and external rotation are the common deformities. A fixed flexion deformity is best determined by performing Thomas's test. Hugh Owen Thomas described this test in 1876. A patient with a fixed flexion deformity at the hip will compensate, when lying on his back, by arching the spine and pelvis into an exaggerated lordosis. A hand placed under the back will assess the lumbar lordosis. If the hip not being measured is flexed to its limit the pelvis rotates and the lordosis is eliminated. During this manoevre the other hip, if in fixed flexion, is passively lifted from the couch. The angle through which it is raised is the fixed flexion deformity (**Figure 6**). An alternative way of assessing fixed flexion deformity is to start with both hips in the knee chest position. Each hip can be extended separately and the angle from the horizontal to the thigh is the flexion deformity.

Extension

Extension is best measured in the prone position with the knee either flexed or straight. Maximum extension is achieved when the pelvis begins to rotate. The normal range is reported to be from 0° to 15–30°.

The main hip extensor muscle is gluteus maximus with contributions from the hamstrings. Power of gluteus maximus is best assessed by asking the patient to lift the leg of the couch with the knee flexed. This minimises the effect of the hamstring muscles.

Abduction

Hip abduction is measured with the patient lying supine and the pelvis stabilised with the examiner's hand on the opposite anterior superior iliac spine. Normal ranges are from 0° to 40–45°. False abduction is detected when the contralateral anterior superior iliac spine moves.

Abductor power is assessed by one hand stabilising the pelvis whilst the other applies resistance to the lateral thigh as the patient abducts. Alternatively, with the patient lying on the side, he or she can be asked to abduct against resistance. Flexing the knee relaxes the iliotibial band and isolates the abductors. An abduction deformity is present when the angle between the transverse axis of the pelvis and the limb is greater than 90°.

Abduction in flexion is often the first movement to be restricted in osteoarthritis of the hip. The patient flexes his hips and knees by drawing the heels towards the buttocks. The knees are then allowed to fall away towards the couch. The normal range is approximately 70°.

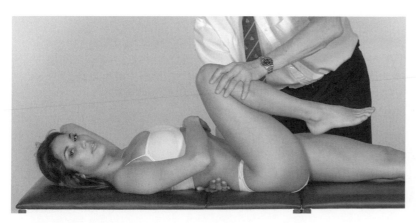

Figure 6 Thomas's Test for a flexion deformity of the hip. The hand placed under the lumber spine confirms the lumbar lordosis has been eliminated. Any persistent elevation or flexion of the thigh relative to the examination couch represents the flexion deformity.

Adduction

True adduction can only be measured if the contralateral leg is in a position of abduction. If it is in a neutral position then a degree of pelvic tilt comes into play as the examined leg crosses over the contralateral static leg. As with abduction, the pelvis needs to be stabilised when measuring the range of movement.

Adductor power is measured by resisting adduction of the abducted leg in the supine position. The examining hand is placed on the inner thigh.

An adduction deformity is seen when the angle between the transverse axis of the pelvis and the limb is less than 90°.

Rotation in extension

Internal rotation is considered normal if the hip rotates from 0° to between 30–40°. External rotation is slightly greater and is recorded from 0° to between 40–60°. It is preferable to use an imaginary line from the patella as opposed the foot to act as a pointer for measurement.

Rotation in flexion

Early signs of hip pathology (e.g. an irritable hip) can be picked up by evaluating rotation in flexion. External rotation is usually greater except in cases of excessive femoral neck anteversion. The range for internal rotation is from 0° to between 30–40° with external rotation from 0° to between 40–50°.

Additional Tests

Rectus femoris contracture

Ely's test is used to evaluate a tight rectus femoris. The patient lies prone and the knee is passively flexed. If the rectus femoris is contracted, then the patient's hip on the same side as the flexed knee will spontaneously rise. Normally the hip will remain flat against the examination couch (**Figure** 7).

Iliotibial band contracture

The Ober test evaluates contracture of the fascia lata or iliotibial band. The patient lies on the unaffected side. The affected hip is extended and abducted. A positive result (i.e. the leg remains abducted) is indicative of a contracture of the iliotibial band. Conversely, a negative result is when the thigh falls to neutral or adduction.

Apprehension test for labral pathology

With the patient supine, the hip is flexed gently, adducted and internally rotated. If this causes pain, there may be an anterior labral tear. An alternative test is the hip apprehension corollary

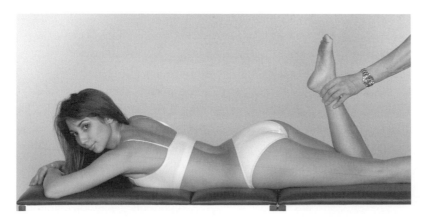

Figure 7 Ely's Test. Passive flexion of the knee in the presence of a tight rectus femoris leads to the ipsilateral buttock rising.

test. The patient lying supine slides down to the end of the table with the affected leg free from support. The leg is brought into extension and external rotation and will cause pain and apprehension if there is labral pathology.

Conclusion

Whether asking the patient to stand or walk before formally examining the hip is not important. It is however, useful to have a standard routine when examining so that you appear competent and no steps are forgotten. Finally having examined the hip, it is important to carry out a vascular and neurological examination of the whole limb.

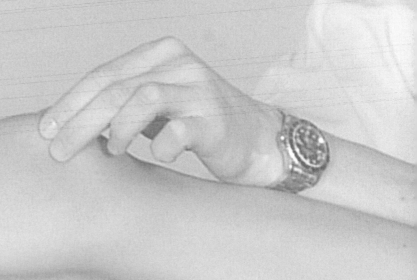

9

Examination of the Knee

D R Bickerstaff

History

General questions

All histories begin with the presenting complaint and, in the case of a joint, the site and side affected. This is then followed by the patient's age, occupation and, specifically in knee related problems, sporting participation (including type and intensity). The latter three are important in ascertaining the patient's degree of functional disability, which clearly has bearing on the range of treatments offered. For instance, a twenty year old professional footballer with an anterior cruciate ligament tear may be offered different advice to a 40 year old office worker who has no active sporting participation but presents with the same injury.

It is then important to ascertain the duration of symptoms, exact details of the precipitating injury, and then the general course of events including response to any treatment already received. It is through this aspect of the history one obtains a clear picture of the degree of disability suffered by the patient.

Usually patients present with a combination of symptoms relating to pain, swelling, locking and giving way, these form the basis of the specific questions asked on taking a history. The diagnostic specificity of each of these symptoms in isolation is poor; rather they are used in combination to guide the examiner to a differential diagnosis. In addition, the presence and degree of each of these symptoms at presentation and then how they changed with the passage of time is important.

Specific questions

Pain

The site of pain within the knee is an indication as to the structure damaged but by no means diagnostic, particularly with traumatic disorders such as meniscal tears. As an example lateral joint pain from a patello-femoral disorder is frequently mistaken for a lateral meniscal tear and, prior to the use of MRI and arthroscopy, resulted in unnecessary lateral meniscectomies. The site of pain following an episode of injury however, such as a medial collateral ligament strain, is a clear indication of the possible structures involved. It is useful to obtain a description of the pain at the time of injury or presentation and then how the pain has progressed. Of particular importance is whether the pain is constant and whether it occurs at night. For instance, these symptoms are an indication to recommend arthroplasty in assessing a patient with severe degenerative changes. Constant pain may indicate more sinister pathology such as tumour or infection.

It is then important to relate the pain to the level and type of activity, such as whether the symptom appears after a few steps walking or only after running. In addition, questions about the pain related to specific actions such as twisting and turning may indicate a problem with the main weight-bearing areas of the knee such as a meniscal tear or chondral defect. Bent knee activities such as kneeling, crouching or squatting may indicate a patello-femoral problem though posterior horn tears of the medial meniscus are aggravated by loaded bent knee activities such as coming up from a squatting position.

The examiner should always be aware of the possibility of referred pain from the hip or lumber spine, particularly when assessing a patient with degenerative symptoms.

Swelling

Swelling can be localised, such as a lateral meniscal cyst, or generalised, such as a haemarthrosis. With regard to local swellings it is important to ascertain the length of time the swelling has been present and whether it is increasing in size and painful. Localised swellings such as bursae, meniscal cysts and ganglia may vary in size, sometimes associated with activity levels, and are common findings. Swellings, which are constant and increasing in size, should be investigated as a matter of urgency, soft tissue or bony tumours around the knee are rare but well reported. Some swellings, such as popliteal cysts, are associated with a generalised effusion and respond to treatment for the generalised inflammation.

Generalised swellings are effusions secondary to an inflammatory process. The commonest effusion is related to some mechanical derangement within the knee such as a meniscal tear or chondral damage. There is usually a history of injury with the effusion appearing within 24 hours. Effusions also occur secondary to inflammatory arthropathies and can be massive if chronic. There is usually no record of injury but a careful history should be taken to identify other features of Rheumatoid arthritis or seronegative arthropathies. These generalised swellings may not be pure effusions; at least part of the swelling may be synovial hypertrophy, which will become apparent on examination if suspected from the history.

Generalised swelling may be secondary to a haemarthrosis, which is generally defined as swelling appearing within 4 hours of an injury. The main differential diagnosis of a haemarthrosis is an anterior cruciate ligament (ACL) rupture, an osteochondral fracture (often associated with a patella dislocation) or a peripheral meniscal tear. Indeed, if an athlete gives a history of a twisting injury on the sports field followed by swelling within 4 hours, they have a 70–80% chance of having sustained an ACL rupture (1). The commonest misdiagnosis in this setting is to confuse an ACL rupture with a lateral patella dislocation, indeed rarely; both can occur together (2). Both occur on the slightly flexed weight-bearing knee forced into external rotation. This reinforces the need for a skyline radiograph in the acutely injured knee to identify a possible osteochondral fragment from the patello-femoral joint that occurs in patella dislocation. This injury is best treated by early re-attachment.

Not surprisingly, haemarthoses are painful due to the degree of tension within the knee. A relatively painless haemarthrosis or diffuse swelling rather than true haemarthosis should alert the examiner to the possibility of a more extensive ligamentous injury with disruption of the capsule. The examiner can be lulled into thinking the injury is less severe than is the case.

Locking

Locking can be subdivided into true locking and pseudo-locking. True locking is relatively rare. It occurs when an intra-articular structure, loose body or meniscal tear interposes between the femoral condyle and tibial surface. Classically the patient can loses terminal extension but is able to flex the knee (though usually also losing some terminal flexion which is less noticeable). They may present with the knee locked but more commonly are able to unlock the knee with a trick manoeuvre involving rotation of the tibia. When the knee unlocks it usually occurs with a clunk and full movement is immediately restored. Loose bodies may also be felt by the patient in the supra-patella pouch but more commonly in either the medial or lateral gutter. They are classically elusive and once found immediately move to another area, hence their eponym of "joint mouse".

Pseudo-locking is a far more common presentation, and usually occurs in patients with anterior knee pain secondary to some form of patella maltracking. Classically it is associated with marked pain and the knee is solidly locked. Over a period of time, often hours, the knee movement gradually returns. The patient usually rests the knee and may use massage and analgesia until the pain subsides. Often this type of locking occurs during some form of bent knee activity, frequently when coming down stairs.

Giving way

There are two types of giving way; true giving way which is usually associated with some form of ligamentous instability, and a buckling type sensation which is usually associated with anterior knee pain and the symptom of pseudo-locking previously described.

An example of true giving way is seen in ACL instability. The patient has no problem running in a straight line but on planting the foot and twisting with the upper body internally rotating, the knee suddenly collapses quickly followed by pain and later swelling. With the initial rupture there may be contact but in the chronic cases this is often not the case. Indeed, in chronic cases, the knee may collapse in actions of every day living. Once the swelling settles the knee apparently returns to normal until the knee gives way again. Again, it is worth bearing in mind the similarity between the symptoms of giving way in chronic ACL rupture and chronic patella dislocation or subluxation (2). If the patella spontaneously reduces and the patient cannot recall the position of the patella, the diagnosis can only be made by careful examination for stability.

Instability from chronic medial instability usually presents with difficulty performing cutting movements rather than rotation. Isolated posterior cruciate ligament (PCL) rupture does not usually present with instability unless there is associated postero-lateral or postero-medial instability. In these situations the knee again feels unstable with rotatory movements but also on walking downstairs due to the unimpeded anterior displacement of the femur on the tibia. Often, patients with these complex problems present with marked instability with active daily living and may constantly need the use of a knee brace.

Buckling of the knee is seen in patients with anterior knee pain and is associated with pain. These patients often report their knee buckling without any rotary movement, usually occurring when walking in a straight line or down stairs. The knee buckling is rarely associated with an effusion.

General Examination

Examination of the knee should follow the usual orthopaedic routine of inspection, palpation, movement and measurement. Specific tests for patello-femoral pathology and stability will also be addressed. One must always remember to use the opposite limb for comparison and to gain the patients trust leave any possible painful tests to the end. A tense patient will make any assessment of subtle instabilities impossible.

The examination should start immediately the patient enters the clinic to assess their gait, walking aids and general mobility. To fully assess the patient however, they should be undressed from mid-thigh, shorts are ideal.

Inspection

Initial inspection should begin with the patient standing to assess over-all limb alignment (**Figure 1**) and any shortening which can be assessed at this stage. Limb alignment includes any femoral or tibial rotational mal-alignments which has a bearing particularly on patello-femoral function. In addition the foot position should be assessed for evidence of any abnormalities such as hyperpronation which again can affect patello-femoral function. It is easier at this stage to assess the posterior aspect of the knee for scars, swellings or bruising. The anterior aspect can be assessed at this stage or later when the patient is supine.

The next step is to observe the gait pattern. There should be sufficient room to watch the patient walking both towards and away from the examiner.

The patient is now laid supine on the examination couch with their head relaxed on a pillow and their hands placed on their chest (**Figure 2**). A patient straining to watch an examination may increase muscle tone affecting observations such as knee laxity. As well as inspecting the anterior aspect of the knee for scars, swellings or bruising, any quadriceps or calf wasting can be observed and measured if thought appropriate. Sometimes swellings, such as lateral meniscal cysts, are best seen with the knee bent to 90° and in comparison with the opposite knee. With the knees flexed in this position they should be observed from the side to identify any posterior sag indicative of a posterior cruciate ligament rupture (**Figure 3**). A prominent tibial tubercle as seen in late Osgood-Schlatters disease may make this assessment difficult.

Palpation

Palpation of the patella and associated structures will be dealt with later. There are two basic tests for the presence of an effusion. The first is balloting the patella on the femoral trochlea having first emptied the medial and lateral gutters of synovial fluid (**Figure 4**). The second is stroking the lateral gutter to empty the fluid and watching for a fluid wave in the medial gutter. If there is the appearance of swelling in the knee and yet no effusion one must consider synovial hypertrophy as seen in conditions such as pigmented villo-nodular synovitis (3).

The knee is largely subcutaneous apart from posteriorly, and as such many structures can be palpated directly. This is best done with the knee bent up to 90° with the foot firmly planted on the examination couch in a neutral position. The fingers can then be

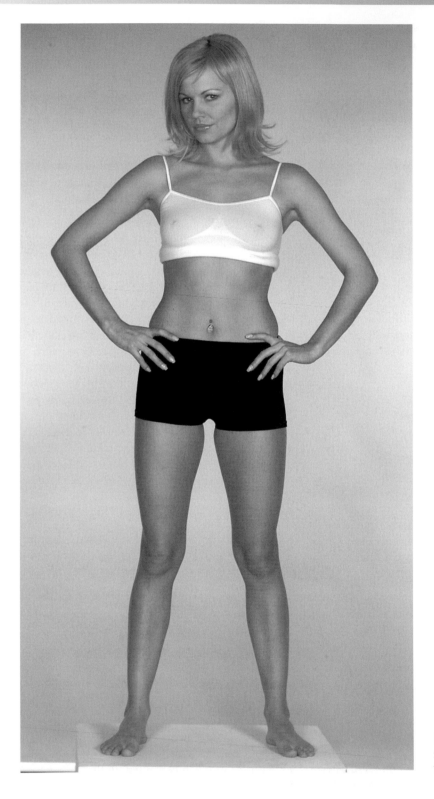

Figure 1 With the patient standing, coronal alignment of the knees is assessed.

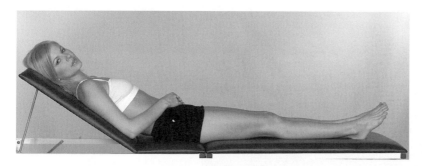

Figure 2 The patient is laid supine in a relaxed position with their hands placed across their chest.

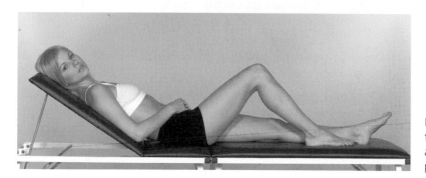

Figure 3 Lateral inspection of the flexed knee will demonstrate a posterior sag, which indicates posterior cruciate laxity.

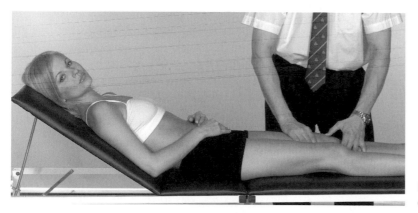

Figure 4 Testing for a knee effusion by balloting the patella.

used to palpate along the joint lines starting with the painless side. Tenderness along the joint line, particular postero-medially, may indicate a meniscal tear. The borders of the femoral and tibial condyles, the patella tendon, and medial (MCL) and lateral (LCL) collateral ligaments can also be palpated for tenderness.

The site of tenderness is important in an MCL strain. Most commonly there is tenderness on the medial epicondyle at the site of the femoral origin of the MCL. This can be confused with disruption of the medial patello-femoral ligament seen in lateral patella dislocation. Tenderness along the medial joint line in an MCL strain is indicative of disruption of the deeper fibres and suggests a potentially more complicated injury. Disruption of the tibial insertion of the MCL and hence tenderness in this area is usually only seen in a major knee injury such as dislocation.

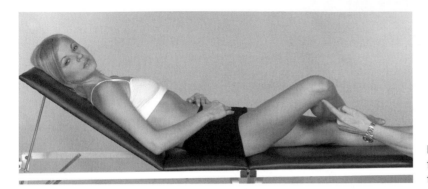

Figure 5 The leg is placed in a figure of four position to palpate the lateral collateral ligament.

The best way to isolate the lateral collateral ligament to differentiate tenderness on the joint line from the tendon itself is to put the patient's leg in a figure-of-four position (**Figure 5**). This puts the ligament under tension making it more pronounced and easier to palpate.

The patella tendon should be palpated in full extension and when tensed at 90° of flexion. In chronic patella tendinosis, tenderness in the proximal tendon is more noticeable in extension, in flexion the normal superficial fibres cover the damaged deep fibres resulting in less pain on palpation.

The posterior aspect of the knee should also be palpated to identify soft tissue masses in the popliteal fossa, which may not have been evident on inspection.

Movement

The assessment of movement relates to active and passive movement of the joint and abnormal movement due to ligament instabilities.

The normal range of passive movement is assessed comparing both sides and including hyperextension. When performing this movement the hand should be placed over the patella to assess the presence and type of patello-femoral crepitus. The range can be noted as degrees of movement such as −10 _ 0 _ 140. Alternatively, hyperextension can be measured as the distance the heel can be lifted of the examination couch and flexion by the heel to but-

tock distance. The patient should be asked to actively perform a straight leg raise to assess the integrity of the extensor mechanism and flex the knee as far as possible.

Measurement

Knee function is obviously affected by any leg length discrepancy. The techniques for assessing this are mentioned in the chapter on hip examination.

Specific Examination

This section will deal with meniscal and patello-femoral pathology and ligament instability.

Meniscal pathology

McMurray's test was to recreate displacement of a meniscal tear which is painful and probably not in the patient's best interests. A modification of this is a compression test to produce discomfort along the joint line, which may indicate pathology in the medial or lateral compartment. The patient is supine with the knee flexed. The examiner places one hand on the top of the knee with the fingers and thumbs positioned to palpate the joint line and the other under the heel (**Figure 6**). The examiner can then compress the joint by pushing down on the top hand while the lower hand controls flexion and can also rotate the leg thereby stressing each compartment in varying degrees of flexion. This test is most

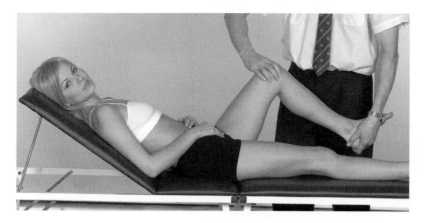

Figure 6 A modification of McMurray's test applies compression to the joint at varying degrees of flexion.

specific for a tear of the posterior horn of the medial meniscus. The patient reports discomfort on the postero-medial joint line with the knee compressed in full flexion and external rotation.

Another less specific test is to ask the patient to fully squat, and if possible duck walk. This action compresses the posterior horns of the menisci but can also cause patello-femoral pain.

No one test for meniscal pathology is absolutely diagnostic (5,6). One usually makes a diagnosis from the history and look for confirmatory tests on examination. The absence of positive signs does not definitely exclude a meniscal tear but other investigations such as a MRI scan should be undertaken.

Patello-femoral pathology

The commonest patello-femoral pathologies include maltracking, which manifests in pain, subluxation or frank dislocation and osteo-arthritis.

An assessment of the overall alignment of the leg including rotational mal-alignment and abnormal foot position has already been mentioned.

With the patient supine and observed in both extension and flexion an assessment of the patella size, position (laterally displaced) and height is made though this is done more accurately with radiographs. The patella is then observed with the patient passively then actively flexing and extending

the knee to observe patella tracking. This is often easier done with the patient's knee flexed over the end of the couch. Rarely one can identify a sudden jerk of the patella as it moves from its laterally placed position into the trochlea at the onset of flexion. Medial displacement of the patella is extremely uncommon and usually iatrogenic. With the leg in this position the patient can then be asked to extend against resistance to induce pain with concentric loading and also slowly allow the leg to flex with the examiner forcibly flexing the knee against a quadriceps contracture to assess eccentric loading.

With the patient supine, the borders of the patella and the retinaculae are carefully palpated for tenderness. In acute patella dislocation, there is a boggy feel to the medial retinaculum with tenderness along the medial border of the patella or over the medial epicondyle at the site of insertion of the medial patello-femoral ligament. With chronic anterior knee pain from mal-tracking there may be tenderness over the supero-lateral border of the patella.

An assessment should then be made of lateral retinacula tightness which one finds with patella tilting such as seen in excessive lateral pressure syndrome. To do this the patella should be just engaged in the femoral trochlea. The knee is flexed slightly by placing one hand balled into a fist under the knee while the other moves the patella maximally medially and laterally (**Figure 7**). If one imagines the patella split

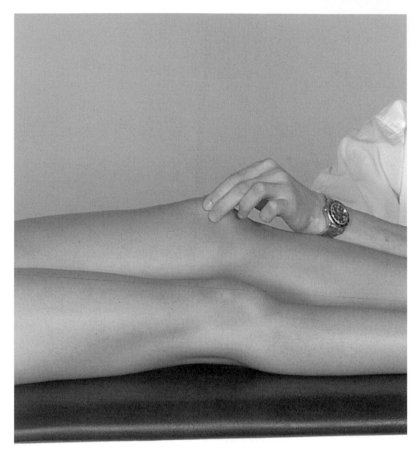

Figure 7 Examining the medial and lateral movement of the patella with the patella just engaged in the femoral trochlea.

into quadrants, the patella should be able to move at least one quadrant medially, any less indicates lateral retinacula tightness. The medial retinaculum is naturally more lax but movement of greater than two quadrants laterally indicates laxity in the medial retinaculum which one may see in recurrent patella dislocation. With the patella held in this lateral position, the knee is now flexed and the patient's reaction observed. A positive patella apprehension test is seen when the patient resists further flexion for fear of the patella dislocating.

Ligament instability

This will be split into three sub-sections, anterior cruciate ligament (ACL) instability, medial collateral ligament (MCL) instability and posterior cruciate ligament (PCL) instability including postero-lateral rotatory instability (PLRI).

ACL instability

Prior to assessing ACL or PCL instability, both knees are viewed from the side when flexed to 90⁰ to identify any posterior sag indicating PCL instability. If this is not recognised, anterior movement from an abnormally posterior placed tibia may be misinterpreted as anterior instability.

The classic test for ACL instability is the Lachman test (7). With a normal sized knee the best technique is to grasp the distal femur with one hand holding the femur still while flexing the knee to 20° and then the other hand grasps the proximal tibia and displaces the tibia anteriorly (**Figure 8**). The amount of

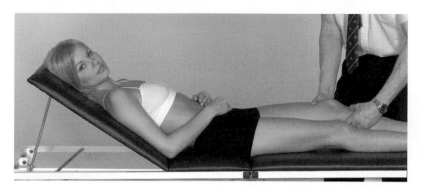

Figure 8 The Lachman test demonstrates anterior displacement of the tibia on the femur at 20° of flexion indicating anterior cruciate ligament rupture.

anterior displacement is then estimated and can be graded. One method of grading is: grade 0 0–3mm (normal), grade I 3–5mm, grade II 5–10mm, grade III >10mm with no endpoint. These measurements are estimated on comparison with the uninjured knee. The amount of displacement is subjective and while useful to the same examiner with subsequent examinations is of little use to another examiner. True measurement of displacement is better undertaken with some form of laxity measurement device though even these are subject to inter-observer error. Of more importance on examination is whether there is definite anterior displacement and whether there is a soft or hard end point. A soft end point is indicative of a complete rupture.

In patients with large thighs or examiners with small hands it is better to fix the femur over the examiners flexed knee while displacing the tibia with the other hand (8).

The other classic test for ACL instability is the pivot shift test (9), which can be performed a number of different ways though the basic principle is the same. The pivot shift test recreates the antero-lateral subluxation of the tibia on the femur which results in the giving way sensation experienced by the patient when twisting on a planted foot. The patients leg is held in full extension with the hands around the knee and the foot tucked under the arm. The lower leg is then internally rotated by twisting the examiners body and a valgus strain applied to the knee via the laterally placed hand and the elbow

and body. In this position, the tibia is antero-laterally subluxed. The knee is then flexed gently and at about 20° the tibia suddenly reduces which can be seen in obvious cases (usually under anaesthetic) and palpated by the hands around the knee in more subtle cases. The degree of instability is increased if the hip is abducted as this decreases tension in the ilio-tibial band (10). It is not possible to perform this test with medial instability, as the medial pivot is lost. The key to this test is obtaining the patients confidence as if performed too forcibly can be distressing for the patient. With the leg securely held and the hands around the knee the patient feels more confident allowing this test to be performed gently and quickly.

Medial collateral instability

This is the commonest form of knee instability. In the acute situation the patient guards the knee and although an impression of medial instability may be gained, the extent of the instability is difficult to assess. In the chronic setting the examination is much easier. The knee is held in the same manner as for performing the pivot shift test. Indeed it is my usual practice to assess collateral stability after the Lachman test and immediately before the pivot shift test, leaving the latter potentially more distressing examination until the end.

With the leg held as described (**Figure 9**) the knee is placed in full extension including hyperextension. A valgus force is then applied to the knee by pushing

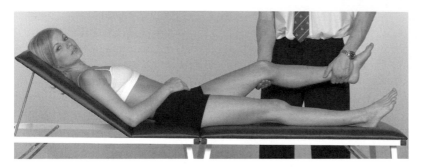

Figure 9 The leg is held to perform a valgus stress test with the foot braced and a valgus force applied to the knee.

the lower leg held by the elbow and body against the laterally placed hand. The degree of opening can be assessed as described in the Lachman test but the most important point is whether there is a soft or hard endpoint. If there is no endpoint with the leg in full extension, this signifies a major disruption of the knee with damage to the cruciate ligaments, which act as secondary stabilisers to valgus strain. Some opening with an endpoint may be present with disruption of the deep fibres of the MCL.

The test is then performed in 20° of flexion, which relaxes the secondary restraints and allows an assessment of the superficial fibres of the MCL. Again an assessment is made as to the degree of movement and the presence of an endpoint.

Postero-medial rotatory instability is a major instability involving damage to the postero-medial structures of the knee (11), principally the posterior oblique ligament, and occurs with severe ligament disruptions, usually affecting the PCL. As well as medial opening in extension and flexion, the posterior subluxation of the medial tibial plateau off the femur can be demonstrated using a "dial test" which is described in the section on postero-lateral instability.

Lateral collateral instability in isolation is unusual and associated with postero-lateral instability, which will be described in the next section. Essentially however, the test is the same as for the MCL. There is greater normal laxity in the lateral structures and care should be taken to compare movement with the uninjured knee.

Posterior cruciate and postero-lateral rotatory instability

These two instabilities are described together as they frequently co-exist but also because there are subtle differences in differentiating the two on examination. The examination for these instabilities should take place concurrently (12) (**Table 1**).

Table 1 Clinical tests in posterior cruciate ligament (PCL)/ postero-lateral corner (PLC) instability			
	PLC	PLC + PCL	PCL
Posterior sag at 90°	N	SP	SP
Posterior draw at 90°	N	SP	SP
Posterior draw at 20°	P	SP	N
Quadriceps active test	N	SP	SP
Valgus stress test	P	P	N
Passive external rotation at 30°	P	SP	N
Passive external rotation at 90°	P	SP	N

As described earlier, before cruciate ligament examination, both knees are flexed to 90° with the patient supine and both feet planted on the examination couch (**Figure 3**). In the posterior sag test, gravity displaces the tibia relative to the femur indicating a PCL disruption.

One then proceeds with the posterior draw test with the knees in this position and the feet planted in neutral rotation. The examiner sits on the feet with hands around the knee (**Figure 10**), the fingers can ensure the hamstrings are relaxed and the thumbs can palpate the joint line. At this angle of flexion the anterior tibial condyles should be anterior to the corresponding femoral condyles. The injured knee is compared with the normal knee and the posterior translation is measured as described earlier in the Lachman test. Another method of grading is grade I if it is 0–5mm (tibia still anterior to the femur), grade II if 5–10mm (tibia flush with femur) and grade III if over 10mm with no end point (tibial condyles sagging behind femoral condyles). In the PCL deficient knee, the posterior draw test at 20°, or "posterior Lachman test", is also mildly positive but more strongly positive in the presence of postero-lateral rotatory instability.

In the quadriceps active test, the patient is positioned as previously. Anterior translation of the proximal tibia with quadriceps contraction indicates a PCL injury.

Although there are many tests described to diagnose postero-lateral instability, I rely on three basic tests. The first has already been described, the "posterior Lachman test". This is most positive in combined PCL and PLRI, slightly less in isolated PLRI and least in PCL instability.

The varus stress test is performed in positioning the patient in exactly the same way as the valgus test described in the MCL section but with a varus force applied to the knee in full extension and 20° of flexion. Increased opening in flexion indicates injury to the LCL, which is usually associated with damage to the postero-lateral corner. Increased opening in extension may still be present in an isolated injury to these structures but is more obvious when combined with anterior or posterior cruciate instability. Comparison with the normal side is important.

The "dial test" is passive external rotation of the tibia (relative to the femur), with the knee at 30° and 90° of flexion. This is best performed with the patient prone, then the feet indicate the degrees of rotation from neutral (**Figure 11**). In the rare case of isolated PLRI, increased external rotation is noted at 30⁰ but less so at 90°. When combined PCL and PLRI are present, increased external rotation is noted in both positions (13,14).

Tests such as the external rotation recurvatum test, reversed pivot shift test and a posterior draw test

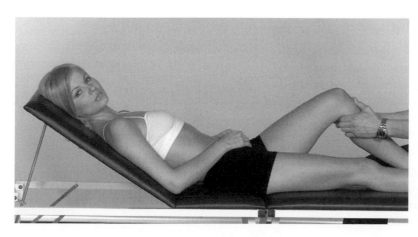

Figure 10 The hands are placed around the knee to palpate the tibial joint line with reference to the femur to assess posterior displacement.

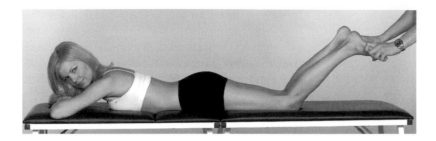

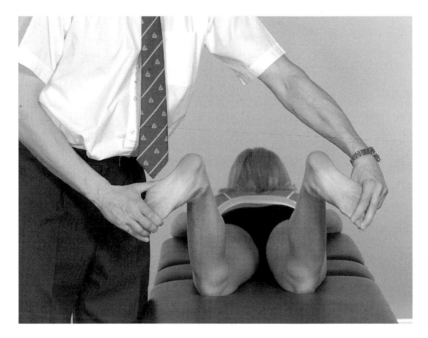

Figure 11 The "dial" test assesses postero-lateral rotation by comparing the injured with the uninjured side with the patient prone.

performed with the foot in external rotation may also be performed for additional confirmation.

Limb alignment and gait pattern must be observed to ensure there is no lateral thrust on walking which is seen in chronic PLRI, usually associated with PCL injury but also seen in ACL injury. If this is not recognised, the ligament reconstructions may fail in the absence of a corrective osteotomy.

PCL and postero-lateral corner injuries are major events and in the acute setting particular care must be taken to ensure there is no neuro-vascular injury, in particular to the common peroneal nerve.

References

1. Maffuli N, Binfield PM, King JB, Good CJ. Acute haemarthrosis of the knee in athletes. A prospective study of 106 cases. J Bone Joint Surg Br 1993; **75(6):** 945–949

2. Simonian PT, Fealy S, Hidaka C, O'Brien SJ, Warren RF. Anterior cruciate ligament injury and patella dislocation: a report of nine cases. Arthroscopy 1998; **14(1):** 80–84

3. Flandrey F, Hughston JC, McCann SB, Kurtz DM. Diagnostic features of diffuse pigmented villonodular synovitis of the knee. Clin Orthop 1994; **298:** 212–220

4. Apley AG, Solomon L. Apley's System of Orthopaedics and Fractures. 6th ed. London: Butterworths, 1982.

5. Stratford PW, Binkley J. A review of the McMurray test definition, interpretation and clinical usefulness. J Orthop Sports Phys Ther 1995; **22(3):** 116–120

6. Evans PJ, Bell GD, Frank C. Prospective evaluation of the McMurray test. Am J Sports Med 1993; **21(4):** 604–608

7. Torg JS, Conrad W, Kalen V. Clinical diagnosis of anterior cruciate ligament instability in athletes. Am J Sports Med; **4(2):** 84–93

8. Draper DO, Schulthies SS. Examiner proficiency in performing the anterior draw and Lachman tests. J Orthop Sports Phys Ther 1995; **22(6):** 263–266

9. Galway HR, MacIntosh DL. The lateral pivot shift a symptom and sign of anterior cruciate ligament instability. Clin Orthop 1980; **147:** 45–50

10. Bach BR Jr, Warren RF, WickiewiczTL. The pivot shift phenomenon: results and a description of a modified clinical test for anterior cruciate ligament instability. Am J Sports Med 1988; **16(6):** 571–576

11. Nielsen S, Rasmusson O, Oveson J, Andersen K. Rotatory instability of cadaver knees after transection of collateral ligaments and capsule. Arch Orthop Trauma Surg 1984; **103(3):** 165–169

12. Miller MD, Bergfeld JA, Fowler PJ, Harner CD, Noyes FR. The posterior cruciate ligament injured knee: principles of evaluation and treatment. Instr Course Lect 1999; **48:** 199–207

13. Staubli HU. Posteromedial and posterolateral capsular injuries associated with posterior cruciate ligament insufficiencies. Sports Med Arth Rev 1994; **2:** 146–164

14. Veltri DM, Warren RF. Posterolateral instability of the knee. J Bone Joint Surg 1994; **76-A:** 460–474.

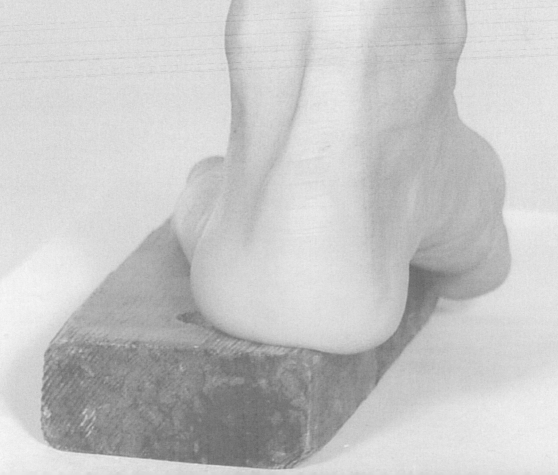

10

Examination of the Adult Foot and Ankle

N J Harris & T W D Smith

History

General

Details of age, sex, occupation and problems with shoewear must always be elicited from patients with foot and ankle problems. Pain, swelling, stiffness, deformity, instability and / or parasthesiae are the usual complaints. Their effects on gait, leisure and employment activities must be clearly established. Many systemic conditions affect the foot. A high index of suspicion must be maintained by clinicians managing foot and ankle disorders. Diabetes, rheumatoid arthritis, seronegative arthropathies, endocrinopathies, gout, pseudogout and vasculitic conditions all directly affect the foot and will influence management strategies. Swelling of the foot and ankle might reflect cardiac, hepatic and renal disease. Unilateral swelling might be the result of secondary obstruction of the lymphatics due to pelvic malignancy especially in women over the age of 50. Lesions of the lumbosacral spine such as a prolapsed intervertebral disc, spina bifida and spinal stenosis may also affect the foot and any history of spinal abnormality must be sought.

Specific

The most important complaint in ankle and foot pathology is pain. Pain referral from primary foot pathology is rare except in entrapment neuropathies. Localization to a specific area therefore narrows the diagnosis significantly. Ankle pain is often felt anteriorly especially in degenerate disease with impingement. Rheumatoid involvement in the ankle is less common than in the other joints of the foot and is usually manifest as a tenosynovitis. Ankle instability presents in two ways, either recurrent sprains or a feeling of looseness when walking on uneven ground or wearing high-heeled shoes. Pain is an uncommon feature unless there is an associated talar lesion. Tarsal coalition may present with ankle instability.

Pain in the subtalar joint is often localised below and behind the malleoli and also in the sinus tarsi. Vanio[1] stated that 60–70% of patients with rheumatoid arthritis will have involvement of the subtalar and mid-tarsal joints. The resulting deformity is one of valgus with patients complaining that the foot is gradually "going over". Tibialis posterior tenosynovitis may exacerbate this.

Heel pain may be localised to either side of the calcaneus especially in conditions such as insufficiency fractures of the calcaneus and Paget's disease. Pain at the insertion of the Achilles tendon and plantar fascia is associated with systemic conditions such as gout, pseudogout and seronegative arthropathies especially when bilateral. Unilateral plantar fasciitis and Achilles tendinitis however usually result from biomechanical and environmental factors, which result in micro-tears and inflammation. Burning pain anterior to the medial calacaneal tuberosity on the plantar aspect of the foot worse with the first few steps in the morning is typical of plantar fasciitis. The presence of a plantar heel spur on X-ray neither confirms nor refutes the existence of plantar fasciitis. Pain located to the insertion of the Achilles tendon made worse with resisted plantar flexion activities is typical of Achilles tendinitis. Pain and swelling posterior to the medial malleolus along the course of the posterior tibial tendon often reflects posterior tibial tendinitis. Any loss of the normal medial arch as in acquired pes planus might also suggest attenuation or rupture of the posterior tibial tendon. Postero-medial pain might also represent flexor hallucis longus tendinitis. Pain of this origin is typically made worse by movement of the hallux. In severe cases triggering of the hallux can occur due to tendon stenosis between the medial and lateral tubercles of the talus. Lateral ankle pain can be caused by peroneal tendinitis and subluxation.

Midfoot pain is less common than hindfoot and forefoot pain. Post-traumatic, degenerative and inflammatory arthritic conditions can all lead to midfoot pain. In the diabetic patient a red, warm painful midfoot without symptoms and signs of infection especially at the cunieform-metatarsal joint is typical of a diabetic Charcot neuroarthopathy.

Forefoot pain or metatarsalgia has many causes. It is simplified by initially establishing whether the patient has an associated callosity or not and secondly whether the patient has neuritic symptoms[2]. **Table 1** outlines a simple algorhythm to help in

Table 1 Metatarsalgia

	Metatarsalgia	
Callosity	**No callosity**	
	Neuritic symptoms	No neuritic symptoms
Hallux valgus	Morton's neuroma	MTP instability
Bunionette	Tarsal tunnel syndrome	MTP capsulitis
Claw, Hammer, Mallet toe	PID	Stress #
IPK		

diagnosis. Patient's with hallux valgus and lesser toe deformities complain of difficulties with shoewear and unsightliness, as well as pain. Symmetrical clawing of the lesser toes and deformity of the hallux is typical of the rheumatoid forefoot. The synovitis causes extension of the metatarsophalangeal joints with subsequent rupture of the volar plate leading to clawing of the toes. The clawed toes pull the plantar fat pad distally and expose the metatarsal heads. Patients describe a feeling of "walking on pebbles". Intractable plantar keratosis (IPK) usually occurs under the 2nd or 3rd metatarsals and is the result of either a transfer lesion because of medial column insufficiency for example such as in hallux valgus or because of problem with the ray itself such as metatarsal overlength. Patients complain of well localised plantar pain directly beneath the metatarsal head on weight-bearing. Nerve compression or irritation can occur at many levels. An accurate history will help localise the pathology. Local lesions can cause narrowing of the tarsal tunnel such as a ganglion, schwannoma or lipoma. Systemic conditions such as myxoedema, must not be forgotten as a cause of nerve compression. Patients with tarsal tunnel syndrome complain of vague diffuse burning pain and tingling over the plantar aspect of the foot which is often worse with exercise. Occasionally, patients complain of pain radiating up the medial aspect of the leg (Valleix phenomenon). In contrast patients with a Morton's neuroma complain of a burning plantar pain well localised between the metatarsal heads. The pain often radiates to the toes of the involved interspace usually the 3rd and 4th. Atypical neuritic symptoms

should alert the physician to more proximal lesions such as a prolapsed intervertebral disc and mononeuritis of diabetes.

Acquired foot deformity in the adult typically presents with pain associated with overloading. The acquired cavo-varus foot has either a neuromuscular or traumatic aetiology (**Table 2**). Patients with a cavo-varus deformity often complain of pain under the metatarsal heads together with lateral instability. They also complain of uneven shoewear in the early stages. The acquired flat foot deformity in the adult often results from posterior tibial tendon dysfunction, rheumatoid disease, trauma, infection or tumour(classically osteoid osteoma). Pain is often felt medially over the prominent talar head and laterally due to impingement of the lateral talar process in the angle of Gissane. Tarsal coalition usually presents in childhood but can present in adults with a fixed planus deformity and ankle instability.

Table 2 Differential Diagnosis of Accquired Cavovarus Foot

Neuromuscular	cerebral palsy
	spinal dysraphism
	spinal cord tumour
	polio
	hereditary motor and sensory neuropathy
	muscular dystrophy
Structural	trauma

General Examination

Inspection

The patient is first examined standing. Many foot and ankle deformities have a neurological basis therefore, from behind the first area to inspect is the lumbar spine for signs suggestive of spinal dysraphism such as a hairy patch, naevus, lipoma, dimple or sinus. Pelvic obliquity or knee skin creases at different levels suggest a leg length discrepancy. The position of the heel in relation to the floor is best assessed from the back, as is any asymmtery of the calves. Swelling of the achilles tendon or posteromedial or posterolateral aspects of the ankle is also best assessed from behind. In this position the relationship between the long axis of the tibia and the long axis of the os calcis should be commented on. This represents the tibiocalcaneal angle and is usually 5° of valgus (**Figure 1**). From behind the patient it is also possible to comment on the amount of the forefoot visible. This has important implications in patients with posterior tibial tendon disruption for example the 'too many toes sign'. From the front the examiner should start with the ankle, commenting on any swelling which might represent synovitis, an effusion or osteophytes. Moving anteriorly the examiner then comments on the medial longitudinal arch. The arch may be flatter than expected (planus) or higher than expected (cavus). There may also be deformity of the midfoot. The forefoot can have many different deformities in the same foot. It is important to describe the deformities in a logical fashion, starting with the hallux and moving laterally. Skin and nail changes must be sought especially in diabetic patients where ulceration is common. Lastly the plantar aspect of the foot must be inspected for evidence of plantar keratoses or ulcers. Diabetic ulcers are typically found under the 1st metatarsal head, the pulp of the hallux and beneath the 2nd and 3rd metatarsal heads.

Palpation

This must again follow a systematic approach starting with the ankle and moving distally. Medially the examiner assesses the ankle for swelling or tenderness which might reflect synovitis or rupture of the posterior tibial tendon, irritation or compression of the posterior tibial nerve or snapping of the flexor hallucis longus (**Figure 2**). Moving anteriorly in a clockwise fashion ankle synovitis or an effusion can be felt in the notch of Harty, which is the space medial to the tibialis anterior. Crepitus might also be felt here with passive movement. Moving laterally the tibilais anterior, long extensors and peroneus tertius can be palpated. As the examiner moves further lateral the anterolateral aspect of the ankle joint can be palpated. Again synovitis, an effusion and crepitus can be detected here (**Figure 3**). From this position the examiner can move superiorly over the inferior tibio-fibular syndesmosis. Tenderness here may reflect injury to this structure. Further tests to support this are the squeeze test where the examiner squeezes the calf at mid-calf level compressing the fibula and tibia in the coronal plane[3] (**Figure 4**). External rotation of the foot with the leg stabilised anteriorly is also a provocative test for syndesmosis injuries (**Figure 5**). Moving distal to the joint line the examiner can palpate the anterior talofibular ligament which runs at an angle of approximately 70° to the long axis of the fibula from the anterodistal aspect of the fibula to the talus. Further anteriorly the sinus tarsi can be palpated. Tenderness here may reflect irritation of the subtalar joint. Moving posteriorly the examiner can palpate the peroneal tendons. The calcaneofibular ligament runs deep to the peroneal tendons creating an angle of approximately 100° with the anterior talofibular ligament. Tenderness in this region may reflect injury to the peroneal tendons, the superior peroneal retinaculum or the calcaneofibular ligament (**Figure 6**). To distinguish between peroneus brevis and longus, the foot is placed in the neutral position and resisted eversion performed (**Figure 7**). This tenses the peroneus brevis which lies anterior to the longus on a line from the lateral malleolus to the base of the 5th metatarsal. To tense the peroneus longus, resisted plantarflexion of the 1st ray is performed (**Figure 8**). Continuing in a clockwise direction the examiner then moves onto the achilles tendon. Tenderness, thickening and nodules can be detected as well as any bony swelling such as in a Haglund's deformity. To distinguish between thickenings of the tendon or tendon sheath passive dorsiflexion and plantarflexion are performed. A thickening of the tendon will

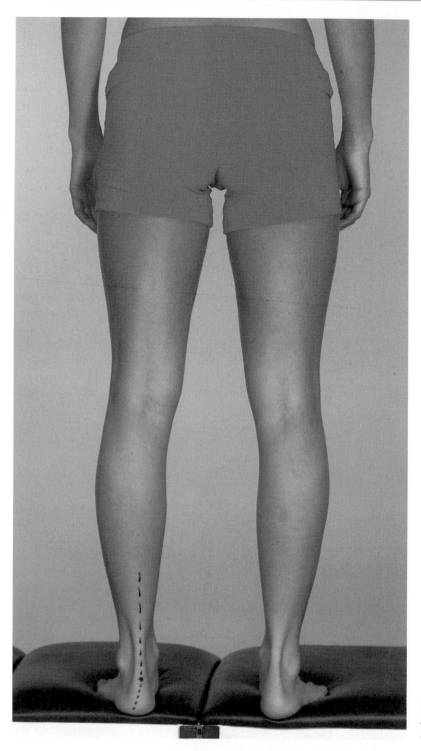

Figure 1 The tibiocalcaneal angle – usually 5° of valgus. *(continued)*

move with movement of the tendon whilst a thickening of the sheath will remain fixed.

Having palpated the ankle the examiner then moves more distally. The calcaneus is the site of origin of the plantar fascia from the antero-medial tuberosity. Tenderness here is indicative of plantar fasciitis (**Figure 9**). Maximally dorsiflexing the great toe tenses the plantar fascia and may provoke further discomfort. This manouvre also recreates the medial longitudinal arch in a patient with a mobile pes planus deformity, the so-called windlass effect (**Figure 10**). The plantar fascia should also be palpated for plantar fibromatoses. Side to side compression of the calcaneus is helpful in identifying patients with structural abnormalities of the heel for example stress fractures (**Figure 11**). Moving distally the examiner then palpates Chopart's joint (talonavicular and calcaneocuboid) for evidence of tenderness and/or crepitus. Between the two joints

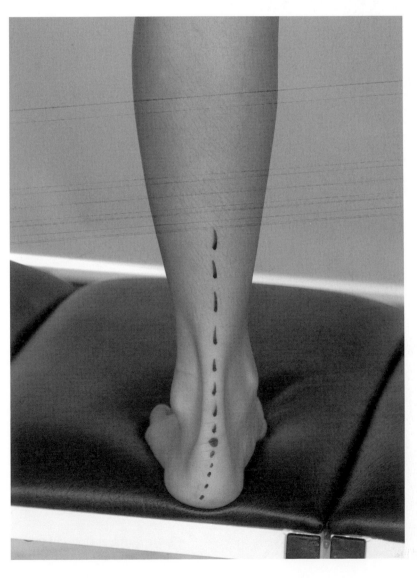

Figure 1 The tibiocalcaneal angle (*close-up*).

is the sinus tarsi, tenderness here is often suggestive of irritation of the subtalar joint. The mid-tarsal joints should be assessed in a similar way. Moving on to the forefoot the examiner starts with the hallux. Tenderness and swelling dorsally at the level of the metatarsophalangeal joint is suggestive of a cheilus associated with hallux rigidus. Tenderness

and swelling along the shaft of a metatarsal especially the second might reflect a stress fracture. Tenderness and swelling of a lesser metatarso-phalangeal joint might reflect a synovitis, such as that associated with Freiberg's disease which typically affects the 2nd metatarsophalangeal joint. Isolated metatarsophalangeal joint synovitis can be detected

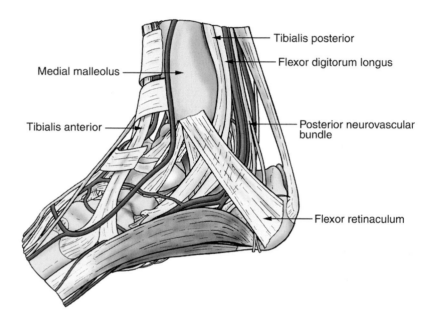

Figure 2 The anatomy on the medial side of the ankle.

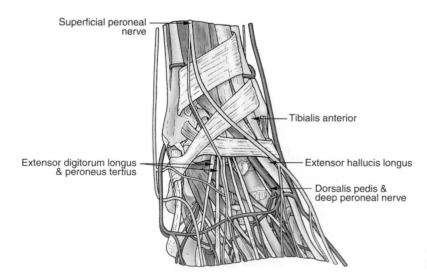

Figure 3 The anatomy of the anterior aspect of the ankle.

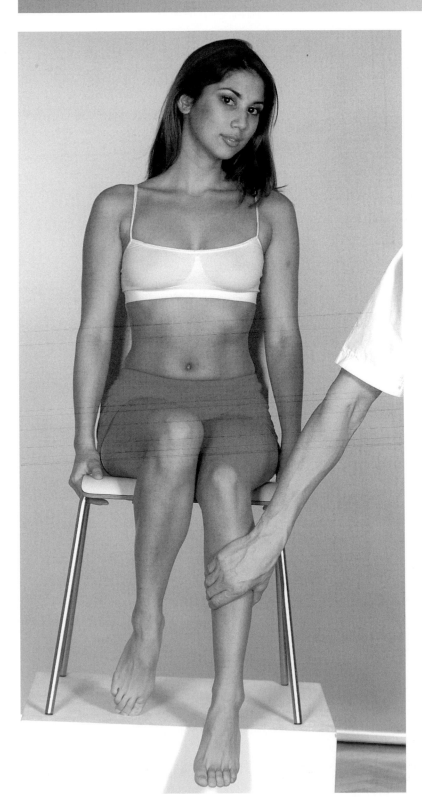

Figure 4 The 'squeeze test' for assessment of the distal tibiofibular syndesmosis.

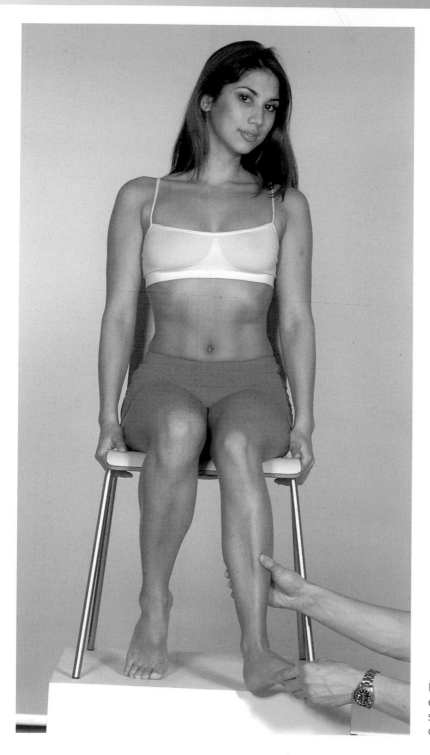

Figure 5 The foot being externally rotated whilst stabilising the leg stressing the distal tibiofibular syndesmosis.

by passively plantar flexing the toes. This manoeuvre is painful in the presence of synovitis. Swelling and tenderness of all the metatarso-phalangeal joints is typical of rheumatoid or psoriatic arthritis. In this case there may be evidence of the 'daylight sign'. Due to the synovitis the toes are pushed apart so daylight can be seen between each. The 'squeeze test' reinforces this. The toes are squeezed in a medio-lateral direction which provokes discomfort if a synovitis is present. Palpation of the plantar aspect of the forefoot attempts to identify specific areas of tenderness often related to plantar keratoses beneath prominent metatarsal heads. Tenderness between the metatarsal heads especially in the 3rd web space and if associated with burning pain and parasthesiae radiating to the toes is typical

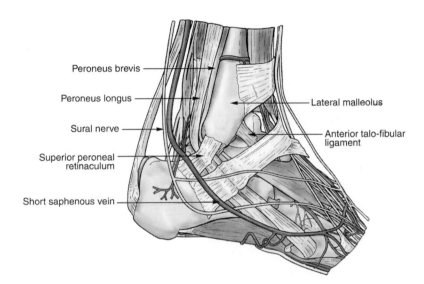

Figure 6 The anatomy of the lateral aspect of the ankle and foot.

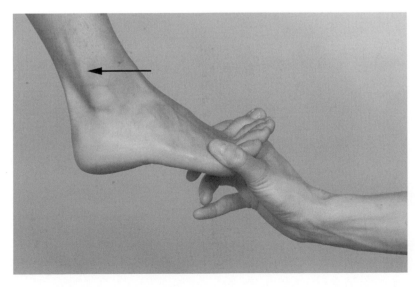

Figure 7 Resisted eversion of the foot stressing the peroneus brevis.

of a Morton's neuroma. Reproduction of the pain when squeezing the toes in a medio-lateral direction and the production of a click by applying dorsally directed pressure from beneath the affected web space further support the diagnosis and is described as Mulder's sign[4] (**Figure 12**) Pain beneath the 1st metatarso-phalangeal joint should alert the examiner to the possibilty of a sesamoiditis either the result of a degenerative process or a stress fracture.

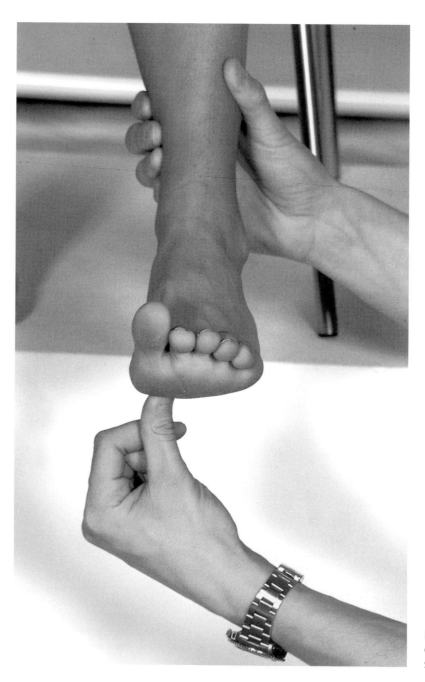

Figure 8 Resisted plantarflexion of the 1st metatarsal which stresses the peroneus longus.

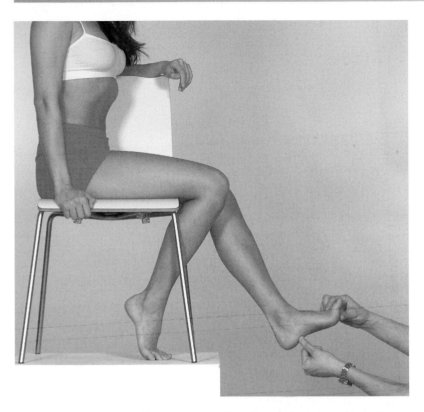

Figure 9 The site of maximum tenderness found in patients with plantar faciitis.

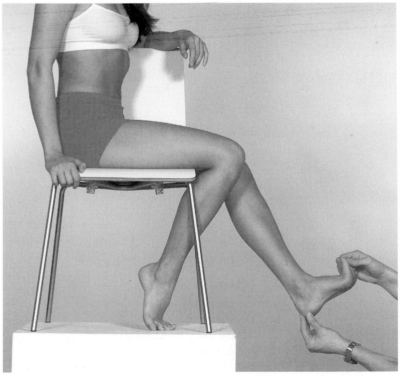

Figure 10 The 'windlass effect'. The great toe is maximally dorsiflexed which tightens the plantar fascia and helps to reform the medial arch.

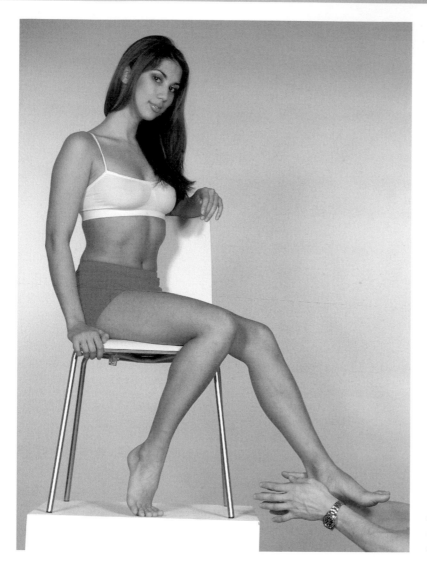

Figure 11 Side-to-side compression of the calcaneus used to identify structural abnormalities of the os calcis.

Movement

This completes the general examination. The standing patient is asked to rise onto tip-toes. This confirms that the gastro-soleus complex is functioning. If both heels adopt a varus position during this manouvre this suggests that both tibialis posterior tendons are functioning as well (**Figure 13**). Active and passive ankle movement is assessed with the patient seated, both with the knee flexed and extended. The usual range of ankle movement is 20° of dorsiflexion and 40° of plantarflexion. Passive movement must be assessed with the forefoot in supination to exclude dorsiflexion at Chopart's and the mid-tarsal joints (**Figure 14**). Inversion and eversion are assessed with the foot in a relaxed position of slight plantarflexion to assess inversion, and a neutral position to assess eversion, remembering that these movements reflect movement not just at the subtalar joint but also at Chopart's and the mid-

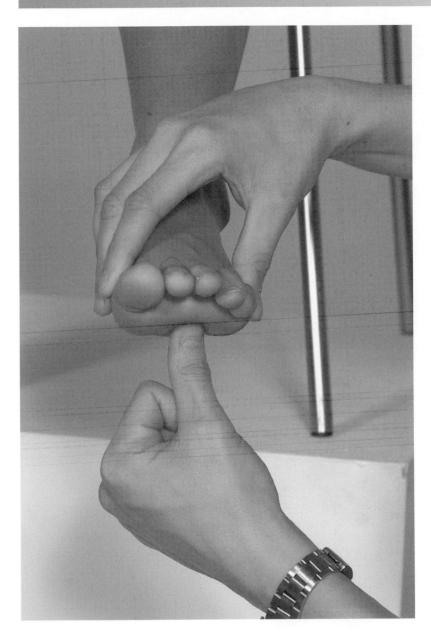

Figure 12 Mulder's Test. The forefoot is being squeezed in a medio-lateral direction whilst at the same time pressure is applied from the plantar aspect of the foot under the affected web space.

tarsal joints. Whilst performing these movements passively, it is possible to assess whether movement is occurring at the subtalar joint or elsewhere in the foot. The amount of inversion is generally twice that of eversion, approximately 20 degress of inversion and 10° of eversion. By fixing the hindfoot the amount of passive pronation and supination occur-ing at Chopart's and the midtarsal joints can be assessed and their contribution to overall inversion and eversion can then be calculated. Subtalar move-ment can be assessed with the foot in a plantigrade position as well. Giannestras[5] stated that in this posi-tion there is only 5° of valgus and 5° of varus move-ment in the subtalar joint . Whilst in this position it

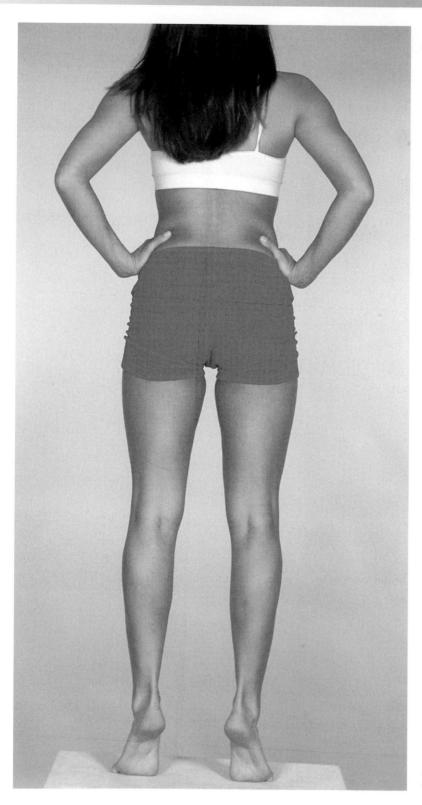

Figure 13 A patient standing on tip-toes with both heels in the normal varus position.

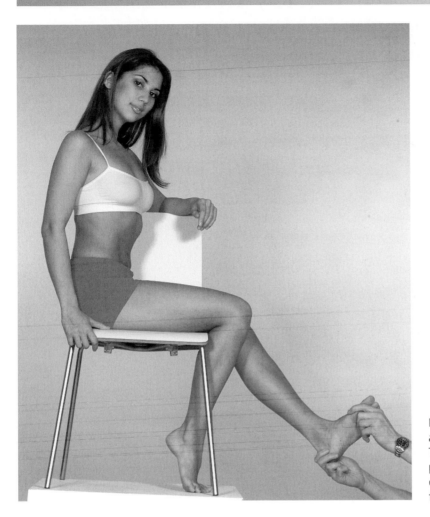

Figure 14 The correct way to assess passive ankle dorsiflexion. The forefoot is supinated to prevent the examiner mistaking dorsiflexion at the the midfoot for ankle dorsiflexion.

is possible to assess the relationship of the forefoot to the hindfoot. With the heel aligned with the long axis of the leg, the thumb of the examiner's hand grasping the heel is placed over the talonavicular joint. With the other hand the forefoot is then repeatedly manipulated until it is felt the talar head is covered by the navicular (**Figure 15**). This is called the neutral position and in this position the relationship of the forefoot to the hindfoot can be commented upon. The forefoot can adopt one of three positions related to the hindfoot, pronated, supinated or neutral. This manoeuvre is of particular value when constructing orthoses, although not commonly performed by most orthopaedic surgeons. Active and passive movement of the hallux is then assessed. The usual range is 80° of dorsiflexion and 40° of plantarflexion relative to the long axis of the 1st metatarsal. In hallux rigidus active and passive movement will be restricted and painful. During passive movement it is often easy to demonstrate impingement between the base of the proximal phalanx and the prominent cheilus on the dorsal aspect of the neck of the 1st metatarsal. A 'grind test' has been described to support a diagnosis of hallux rigidus. The great toe is grasped, loaded and then rotated in the coronal plane. This reproduces the patient's symptoms if there is complete joint involvement rather than isolated impingement.

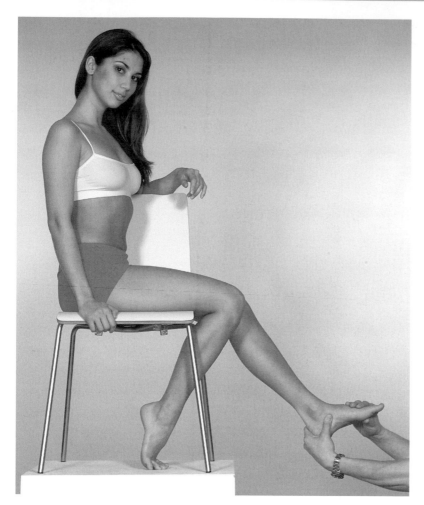

Figure 15 One way of assessing the relationship of the forefoot to the hindfoot with the heel in neutral and the talonavicular joint reduced (side view).

Neurovascular assessment

This is undertaken after the three basic steps of inspection, palpation and movement have been completed. It is important to emphasize that many foot and ankle deformities result from neurological conditions. Inspection of the lumbar spine is therefore an integral part of examination of the foot and ankle. Similarly, in anyone complaining of neurological symptoms in the foot, it is also important to exclude lumbar nerve root tension. Assessment for clonus will distinguish between upper and lower motor neurone lesions. Assessment of sensation will help identify patients at risk for ulceration and will also distinguish between conditions such as polio

and spina bifida, both of which are lower motor neurone lesions. Motor testing should initially assess myotomal function and then concentrate on specific muscle groups as directed by the history and examination. Assessment of the pulses concludes the initial general examination.

Although it is always important to consider the possibility of distant neurological disease affecting the foot and ankle, there are certain entrapment neuropathies around the foot and ankle that can be responsible for numbness, parasthesiae and wasting. Tarsal tunnel syndrome results from compression of the posterior tibial nerve in the tarsal canal. It is characterised by diffuse plantar pain associated with

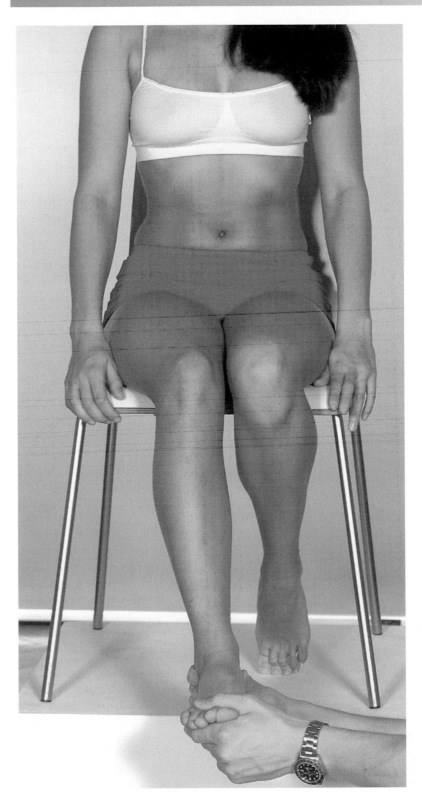

Figure 15 *(continued)* Front view.

parasthesiae and numbness. Percussion over the area of the entrapment may reproduce the symptoms and palpation along the course of the nerve may reveal local causes such a lipoma, ganglion or exostosis. Physical findings must be supported with electrodiagnostic studies especially if surgery is planned. Deep peroneal nerve entrapment occurs most frequently beneath the inferior extensor retinaculum. It is often associated with trauma such as repeated ankle sprains. Patients complain of pain in the dorsum of the foot with radiation into the first web space. Examination may reveal reduced sensation in the first web space and wasting of the extensor digitorum brevis. Superficial peroneal nerve entrapment results from impingement of the nerve on the deep fascia as it exits the lateral compartment approximately 10 cm proximal to the ankle joint. Patients complain of pain in the lateral distal calf often associated with numbness and parasthesiae on the dorsum of the foot. Examination reveals point tenderness where the nerve exits the compartment. Where either deep or superficial peroneal nerve entrapment is suspected the examiner must always palpate the common peroneal nerve around the neck of the fibula. Other entrapment neuropathies have been described such as sural nerve entrapment and entrapment of the first branch of the lateral plantar nerve. These must be considered once more common lesions have been excluded.

Features of Specific Pathological Conditions and Special Tests

Achilles tendon disruption – the patient often describes being struck at the back of the leg. They are unable to perform a heel raise, a palpable gap is felt and when placed supine, squeezing the calf does not produce plantarflexion (Thompson Test[6]).

Peroneal tendon dislocation – results from disruption of the superior peroneal retinaculum. It recurs in more than 50% of cases. In the chronic setting the patient describes a popping or snapping sensation lateral to the ankle. Movement of the foot and ankle from full plantarflexion and inversion to full dorsiflexion and eversion will often reproduce the dislocation. Pain and tenderness over the tendons is suggestive of a concomitant tear of the tendons.

Posterior tibial tendon disruption – results from progressive degenerative change within the tendon. Symptoms range from pain and swelling along the medial aspect of the ankle to postural changes with loss of the medial longitudinal arch and hindfoot valgus. In patients with complete disruption of the tendon more toes are visible when viewing the patient from behind the so called 'too many toes sign'[7] due to increased abduction of the forefoot. When the patient is asked to perform a double heel rise the affected foot remains in valgus rather than shifting into varus as is the usual case. When asked to perform a single heel rise the patient is often unable to do this. To test tibialis posterior function the foot is plantarflexed and everted. From this position resisted inversion is undertaken which stresses the tibialis posterior (**Figure 16**). It is important to assess whether the hindfoot is fixed in valgus or corrects into varus and whether any compensatory forefoot position is fixed or mobile as this affects the treatment options.

Ankle instability can only be diagnosed with certainty using stress radiographs. An inversion stress test is performed with the foot in a relaxed position of slight plantarflexion. The ligament being stressed is the calcaneofibular. Comparison with the other side may reveal a difference but radiographs are needed to define whether the instability is occurring in the ankle, subtalar or both joints. The anterior drawer test assesses the anterior talofibular ligament. In severe cases a suction sign develops just anterior to the lateral malleolus. Again though, radiographs are required to confirm that the instability is occurring in the ankle.

Cavo-varus foot deformities – the commonest cause in the adult is Charcot-Marie-Tooth disease (Hereditary Motor and Sensory Neuropathy type I). It is autosomally dominantly inherited and typically presents in the second decade with symmetrical deformities. Asymmterical cavo-varus deformities are more typical of spinal dysraphism. Patients with Charcot-Marie-Tooth develop hindfoot varus, pes cavus, clawing of the toes and plantarflexion of the 1st ray. Plantarflexion of the 1st ray is the result of

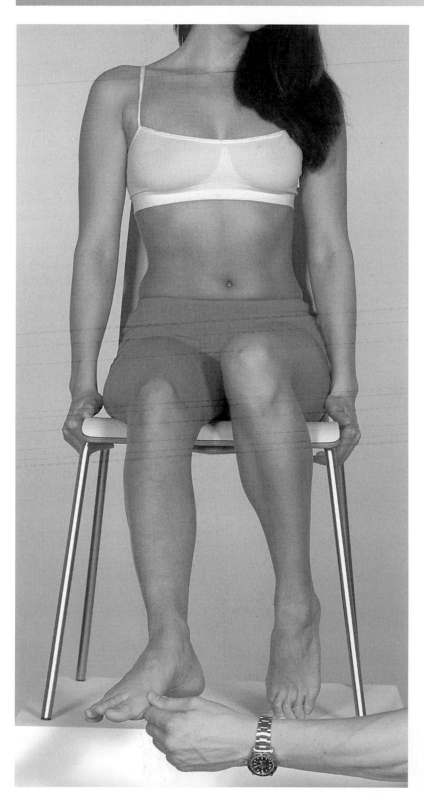

Figure 16 How to assess tibialis posterior power with the foot plantarflexed and everted.

sparing of the peroneus longus. In order to get the lateral four metatarsals plantigrade the heel must move into varus. The examiner must determine whether the hindfoot varus is fixed or mobile. The Coleman Block Test[8] is used to distinguish between the two. A block is placed beneath the foot such that the 1st ray is not supported (**Figure 17**). If the heel is mobile it should adopt a valgus positon. If it remains in a varus position it can be regarded as a fixed defromity.

Tarsal coalition usually presents in children when the fibrocartilagenous bar, which represents a failure of segmentation of the tarsal bones, ossifies. Patients complain of foot fatigue and hindfoot pain. In adults, recurrent ankle sprains may be a presenting feature. Tenderness is detected in the sinus tarsi with a calcaneonavicular bar and medially around the sustentaculum tali with a talocalcaneal bar. The classical description of presentation with a tarsal coalition is one of a 'peroneal spastic flat foot'. The hindfoot is fixed in valgus with no inversion of the foot permitted. Not all patients with a coalition however have a fixed valgus deformity, some have neutral alignment and some a varus deformity. The differential diagnosis of a fixed flat foot deformity in an adult includes septic arthritis, osteoid osteoma, inflammatory arthropathy, trauma and posterior tibial tendon disruption.

Rheumatoid foot has a characteristic pattern of involvement. The hindfoot is often in valgus due to involvement of the subtalar joint and also the posterior tibial tendon. The midfoot is abducted with loss of the medial longitudinal arch. There is clawing of the lesser toes and hallux valgus. On the plantar aspect of the foot there are callosities over the prominent metatarsal heads.

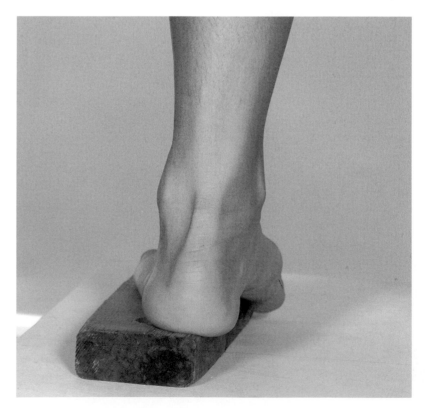

Figure 17 The Coleman Block Test. The medial aspect of the forefoot especially the great toe is placed off the edge of the block allowing the heel to move back into a valgus position if there is no fixed deformity (close-up view).

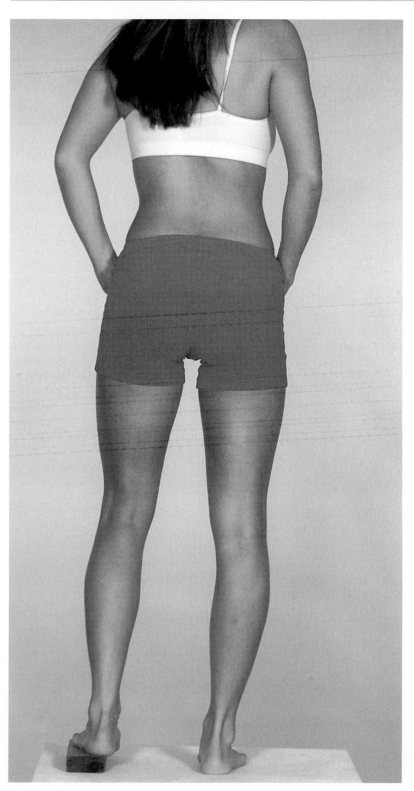

Figure 17 Full view.

Foot and Ankle Terminology

N J Harris & M M Stephens

'There still exists a considerable ambiguity in the use of terms considering the joints of the human foot and their motions despite the efforts toward standardising both of anatomists and clinicians' Huson 1987.[9]

There are several reasons for this. The first is an embryological one. The foot is initially aligned with the leg, but rotates through 90° during development. This causes two of the axes of motion of the foot to do the same (**Figure 18 a, b**). Position and movement of hindfoot are usually described with reference to the axes of motion of the leg whilst the mid and forefoot (distal to Chopart's joint) are described relative to their embryological axes. If internal and external rotation of the mid and forefoot are replaced with pronation and supination there become obvious similarities with upper limb movements.

Another reason for the confusion is that movements of the foot and ankle rarely occur in one plane. Combination patterns of movement have been described as early as 1889 by Farabeuf.[10] In the following text inversion and eversion are used to describe these combination movements. Inversion refers to plantarflexion, adduction and supination of the mid and forefoot together with plantarflexion, adduction and internal rotation of the hindfoot. Eversion is the opposite with dorsiflexion, pronation and abduction of the mid and forefoot together with dorsiflexion, abduction and external rotation of the hindfoot.

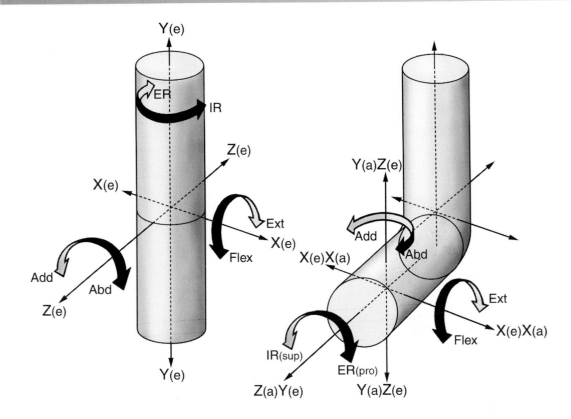

Figure 18 (a) Axes of motion of the embryo. (b) Axes of motion of the adult mid and forefoot. It can be seen how the embryological axes Z(e) and Y(e) have both rotated through 90°, but that the X(e) axis remains constant

References

1. Vanio K. The rheumatoid foot: a clinical study with pathologic and roentgenological comments. *Ann Chir Gynaecol* 1956; **45(supp):** 1–107

2. Coughlin MJ. Common causes of pain in the forefoot in adults. *Journal of Bone and Joint Surgery* 2000; **82(B):** 781–790

3. Hopkinson WJ ,St Pierre P, Ryan JB. Syndesmosis sprains at the ankle. *Foot & Ankle* 1990; **10:** 325–330

4. Mulder JD. The causative mechanism in Morton's metatarsalgia. *Journal of Bone and Joint Sugery* 1951; **33:** 94–95

5. Giannestras NJ. *Foot Disorders: Medical and Surgical Management 2nd Edition*. Lea & Febiger, 1970 Philadelphia.

6. Thompson T, Doherty T. Spontaneous rupture of the tendon of Achilles: a new clinical diagnostic test. *J Trauma* 1962; **1:** 126–129

7. Churchill RS, Sferra JJ. Posterior tibial tendon insufficiency. Its diagnosis, management and treatment. *Am J Orthopaedics* 1998; **27(5):** 339–347

8. Coleman SS, Chestnut WM. A simple test for hindfoot flexibility in the cavovarus foot. *Clin Orthop* 1977; **123:** 60–62

9. From: Sarrafian SK. Anatomy of the Foot and Ankle, 2nd edition. 1993: Lippincott, Philadelphia, USA.

10. Farabeuf LH. *Precis de Manuel Opertoire*: 816–847. Paris. Masson. 1889

11

Orthopaedic Examination Techniques in Children

J A Fernandes & M J Bell

Paediatric orthopaedic examination is an art and the success of the consultation relies on the surgeon's ability to communicate with the parents and the child. Most children referred do not require surgery and time is spent on reassuring the anxious parents or guardian of the normal variations in the development of the child.

The paediatric consulting area should be child friendly with toys and ample space for the child to play and for the surgeon to observe. Gaining confidence from the child is crucial as well as being warm and patient with the parents who are the most anxious and concerned. The initial interview should include introductions' as it's important to know the accompanying adults apart from the parents. They could be carers, guardians, grandparents or physiotherapists as valuable information could be gained. History should be gained from the parents as well as the child, for not infrequently it could be conflicting. Clinical history skilfully obtained is the key to diagnosis and a methodical examination of the child depending on the age and symptoms confirms your initial impressions.

History

General

The history usually starts with some statistical and demographic data, followed by the presenting complaint. Common complaints are of deformity, limp, gait abnormalities, weakness generalized or localized, pain, swelling or stiffness of joints. It's worthwhile asking the older child about his symptoms. The chronological order of the mode of onset, time period, severity, disability, and aggravating and relieving factors should be noted. History of trauma should be investigated thoroughly for it's aetiological significance. Since many of the symptoms arise from the musculoskeletal system that is concerned with support and locomotion, questions should be directed to establishing a relationship of symptoms to physical activity.

Prenatal history is of paramount importance. History of unusual incidents, vaginal bleeding, infection's like rubella in the first trimester give clues in the congenital affections. Maternal history of diabetes mellitus, toxaemia and syphilis are associated with abnormalities at birth. Fetal movements in later pregnancy can be reduced in Arthrogryposis multiplex congenita and Werdnig-Hoffman Disease. In the birth history, the type of presentation, birth weight and Apgar score should be asked for. Further perinatal-related questions including jaundice should be enquired.

Developmental history for physical and mental milestones should be asked for (**Table 1**). Upper limb developmental functions and handedness is important. Information about school performance and physical activities give further insight. This is

Table 1	The important developmental milestones	
Age	**Motor**	**Language**
3 months	Lifts head up when prone	Vocalises without crying
6 months	Head steady when sitting	Smiles and laughs
9 months	Pulls self to stand	Non specific words(da-da,ma-ma)
1 year	Walks with one hand support	Two or more words
14 months	Walks without support	
2 years	Runs forward	Three word sentences
3 years	Jumps in place	Knows whether boy or girl
4 years	Balances on one foot	Counts three objects correctly
5 years	Hops on one foot	Names four colours
6 years	Skips	

usually followed by a systemic review including unusual bruising, easy bleeding and about allergies. Past illnesses, hospitalisations and family history completes the orthopaedic history.

Specific

Limp and gait disturbances

Did the child start limping with complaints of pain? How was the onset? Acute transient synovitis of the hip usually is associated with a history of upper respiratory tract infection 7- 14 days before the episode. The pain could be in the hip, knee or thigh. Was there any history of trauma? Post-traumatic avulsions of apophyses around the hip produce a painful limp. Where is the pain? Adolescent children developing slipped capital femoral epiphyses more commonly present with aching pain around the groin, thigh and often the knee. This may be associated with abnormal gait especially with the chronic slip. In the acute slip, there may be sudden severe pain with difficulty to weight bear. Children in the age group of 4-8 years are more likely to have the

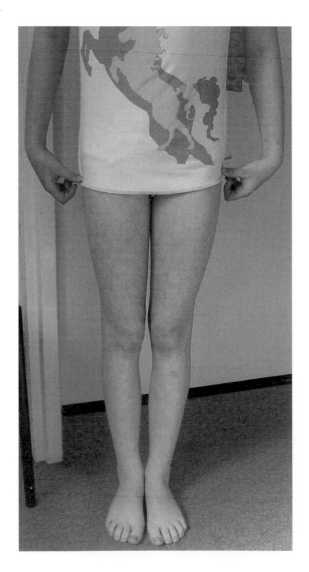

Figure 1 Clinical features for an intoeing type of presentation.

initial presentation of Perthes Disease. Painful limp and difficulty to weight bear with constitutional and systemic symptoms should be urgently assessed for septic affection of joints commonly the hip or in bone.

Was the limp noticed from walking age? Painless limp with short leg could be seen in late presentation of a dislocated hip and painful limp at the end of the day could be a symptom of adolescent acetabular dysplasia. Abnormal asymmetrical gait could be features of a neurological presentation. Abnormal posturing and gait abnormalities might be the only symptoms in rare spinal cord tumours and even in lumbar disciitis.

Deformities

Flexible flatfeet are usually familial with some family history of ligamentous laxity. Is there progressive deformities of toes and feet? Pes cavus warrants a family history to rule out Hereditary Sensorimotor neuropathy or other disorders. Painful flatfeet in adolescence could be the first presentation of tarsal coalitions or inflammatory arthropathies.

In-toeing gait is one of the common complaints (**Figure 1**). If present from walking age and bilateral, usually the common causes are persistent excessive femoral anteversion or internal tibial torsion that does remodel with time. Any unilateral intoeing or out-toeing needs to be further assessed and if rapidly progressing a pathologic condition such as neurologic, tumour, infection and congenital causes should be considered.

Bowlegs and knock-knees are common deformities for which parents ask for consultation. Ask about the progression of these deformities? Quite often they are physiological and if severe need to be further investigated. Nutritional rickets is one of the commonest causes in the developing and third world, whereas questions relating to renal and familial rickets should be asked when such deformities are seen in this Country. Any asymmetric deformity could have an underlying cause. Think of Blount's Disease in an Afro-Caribbean child with tibial bowing.

Limb length discrepancy

Limb length discrepancy, with or without associated deformities, could be due to various causes. When was it first noticed? Was it noticed at birth and is it progressing? Is one shoe size smaller than the other? Is the child using a shoe raise? Does the child complain of any backache? Is one limb larger in length and girth as in hemihypertrophy? Is there a family history of neurofibromatoses? Was there any history of trauma or injury to the growth plates? Was there any history of infection of a joint or bone? These could cause discrepancy with deformity. A positive family history for deformity may indicate a syndrome or some skeletal dysplasias.

Weakness

Localised weakness in the lower or upper limbs are rare and could be due to neuropraxias after injury or due to any bony lumps pressing on nerve structures as in hereditary multiple exostoses. Adolescents could occasionally present with back pain, sciatica and weakness of toe dorsiflexors in acute disc protrusion. Generalised weakness could be a feature of metabolic bone disorders. Boys who complain of easily being tired and toe walkers should be investigated for muscular dystrophy. Neuromuscular conditions like myopathies and others may present with floppy baby, slow developmental milestones, awkward gait and weakness. Space occupying lesions in the base of skull or spinal cord may have unusual presentations of weakness with abnormal gait.

Obstetrical birth palsies can present with deformities, abnormal posture and partial or total loss of movements of the upper limb. Was there a large head or breech presentation? Was there a history of difficult labour? When was it first noticed and is there any progress in recovery of movements?

Swelling

When did the swelling appear and is it getting larger? Is there pain and has it progressed in size rapidly? These could be localized swellings or generalized around joints. Soft tissue swellings usually are slow growing and benign like ganglias and usually pain-free. Any swelling associated with pain should be evaluated for soft tissue sarcomas. Does the swelling fluctuate in size? Haemangiomas, which are common around the knee, give a history of fluctuation in size as well as the semimembranous bursa at the back of the knee. Bony lumps are usually in the metaphyseal regions of the long bones and could be multiple as in Hereditary multiple exostoses. Any associated pain, functional loss, or compromise in joint movement needs to be asked for.

Swelling of joints with associated joint stiffness needs further questioning regarding the onset, periodicity, small or big joints and whether there was a rash or erythematous reaction. Family history of inflammatory conditions should be asked for. Single joint affections need to be further explored for any foci of infection and systemic symptoms like pyrexia.

Scoliosis

History should include whether this was noticed at birth or was associated with any other congenital condition or syndrome. If later, when was it noticed? Is it progressing rapidly and is it associated with other chest cage deformities? Is there any associated pain? Painful scoliosis is a presenting syndrome for an underlying spinal cord or cauda equina tumour as well as bony tumours of the spine such as Osteioid osteoma or Osteoblastomas. Night pain could be an ominous symptom. Ask for family history of Neurofibromatosis? Other neuromuscular conditions like cerebral palsy and Duchennes' muscular dystrophy also develop scoliosis.

Examination

Examination of the child starts from the child entering the room and observing while you take the history. Many clinical signs can be picked up from the parents giving clues in the genetically inherited conditions like neurofibromatosis, flat feet and scoliosis. The child should be undressed appropriately and in stages if required. Babies below the age of 6 months can be examined on the couch and the toddler and infant on the parent's knee until confidence is gained. Respecting the older child's modesty is vital. Examining the orthoses or shoewear may give further information.

General

Inspection of the facies may give valuable clues in syndromic conditions and other skeletal dysplasias. Dysmorphic features when noted need to be of significance and looking at the parents' facies may also help. Blue sclerae can clinch the diagnosis for Osteogenesis imperfecta and mongoloid features for Down's syndrome. The height of the child should be recorded as well as the parents, both standing and sitting. Anthropometric measurements should include head and chest circumference, span, segmental lengths and ratios of the different segments. Any asymmetry in the body proportions of each side including the tongue should be looked for.

Standing examination in general

Examine from the front, side and the back and assess the standing posture and the normal curves of the spine. Look at the level of the shoulders and contour, level of the ASIS and symmetry is looked for. A plumb line held at the center of the occiput should pass thro the natal cleft. Frontal and sagittal balance should be assessed. Look for external spinal markers of dysraphism (**Figure 2**), café-au-lait spots (**Figure 3**), axillary or inguinal freckling, neurofibromas as in neurofibromatosis, any vascular markings as in Klippel-Trenaunay syndrome or other blemishes. Note whether there are any defects of the limbs. If the creases of the limbs are not matching and the pelvis not square, use blocks to lift the shorter side and level the iliac crests.

The general alignment of the lower limbs is then assessed for genu varum or genu valgum (**Figure 4**) and can be quantified with graduated wooden triangles at the intercondylar or intermalleolar levels. The feet should be assessed for any cavus, flat-footedness and hindfoot alignment. Standing on tiptoes should lead to the formation of a nice medial longitudinal arch (**Figure 5**) and the heels should go into neutral or varus (**Figure 6**). The hindfoot should normally be in 7 degree valgus to the long axis of the calf when standing.

Gait

Next ask the child to walk in a straight line and look for any abnormal upper limb movements suggesting

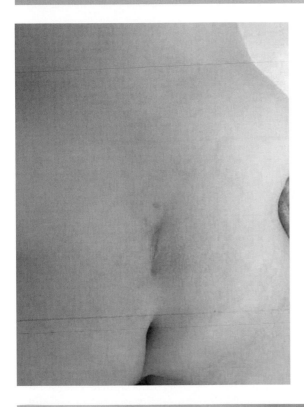

Figure 2 Shows a dimple at the bottom of the spine indicating spinal dysraphism.

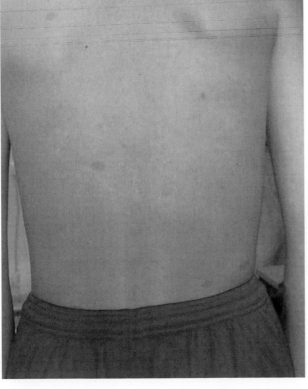

Figure 3 Café-au-lait spots in neurofibromatosis.

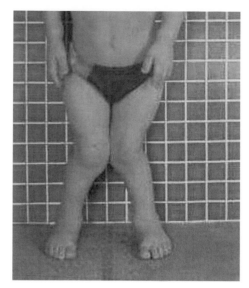

Figure 4 Genu valgum deformity at the knees in *pseudoachondroplasia*.

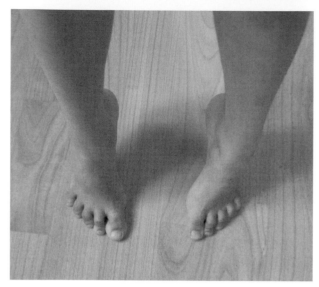

Figure 5 The medial longitudinal arch on standing tiptoes.

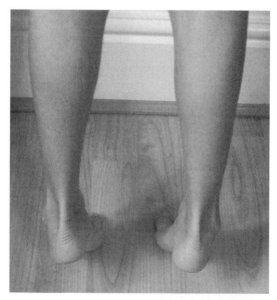

Figure 6 The heels going into varus on standing tiptoes.

hemiplegia, athetoid or spastic movements. Look at the foot progression and knee progression angles, which give the degree of intoeing or outtoeing and the level from where they arise. Look at the way the foot strikes the ground and whether a normal heel to toe type of gait is present. Assess knee extension on heel strike and flexion in swing. Look at the pelvis in all the three planes.

Limp

Can be described as any asymmetrical movement of the lower limbs. They can be due to pain when it's called antalgic or result from limb length discrepancy, instability at the hip or neurological.

An antalgic gait is when the stance phase of the affected limb is hurried with a quick swing phase of the opposite limb. It can be due to any painful cause from the sole of the foot to the pelvis.

Short limbed gait is when the shoulder dips down on the shorter side on stance phase as seen in children with longitudinal deficiencies.

The Trendelenburg gait is due to failure of the abductor mechanism on the affected side to hold the pelvis level in the stance phase with a compensatory sway of the ipsilateral shoulder (lurch) thereby shifting the centre of gravity. This produces a characteristic waddling or swaying, which becomes very dramatic in bilateral affections e.g. bilateral neglected CDH, bilateral coxa vara.

High stepping gait is seen in hereditary sensorimotor neuropathy or when there is ineffective dorsiflexors at the ankle to achieve foot clearance and also produces the slapping foot. This abnormality is seen in swing phase.

The toe walking gait is when the child's initial contact is with the forefoot and the contralateral foot follows the same. When the triceps surae is weak a calcaneus gait is seen with lack of push-off.

The stiff knee produces a limp and the pelvis is either hiked to clear the limb or the patient can circumduct the leg. When the quadriceps is weak, patients compensate by "back kneeing" to prevent the knee from collapsing and fixed equinus helps to achieve this. Some children will use the hand to push the front of the thigh backwards to achieve back kneeing.

Neurological gaits are of various types and can be of combinations. Spastic gait is of equinus at the ankle, flexion at the knee and hips, with adduction and internal rotation of the lower limbs producing dragging or scraping characteristics. Scissoring of the lower limbs can be seen when there are adduction and internal rotation deformities at the hips. The crouch gait is when the triceps is weak and the gait lacks push-off.

Ataxic gait is associated with a broad base and when severe the feet are thrown out producing the double tapping stamping type of gait. Cerebellar ataxias also have a broad based gait, irregular and unsteady with or without eyes open and the child is unable to do tandem walking.

Children with myopathies have a Penguin type of gait and "Gower's sign" is positive where the child uses the hands to climb upon himself to stand up from the sitting posture. The hypertrophied or bulky calves are seen in these boys with wasting of the thigh musculature.

Spine

Assess the primary and secondary curves of the spine from the side. From the back the spine should be straight and any lateral curvature seen is called as scoliosis (**Figure 7**). Any list of the upper body and flank creases should be looked for. Feel the spine for alignment, tenderness, or a step at the lower lumbar spine as in spondylolysistheses.

Forward bending will reveal a structural scoliosis with the development of an asymmetrical rib or lumbar hump (**Figure 8**). Postural or non-structural scoliosis does not show this and can be due to leg length discrepancy or pain due to nerve root entrapment. Scoliosis due to leg length inequality can be corrected by using appropriate blocks and making the pelvis level. Structural scoliosis should be assessed for the type of curve and the level of the curve. The usual curve patterns of single right thoracic, single left thoracolumbar or lumbar are the ones we generally see in adolescent idiopathic scoliosis. The flexibility of the curve should then be assessed by side-bending

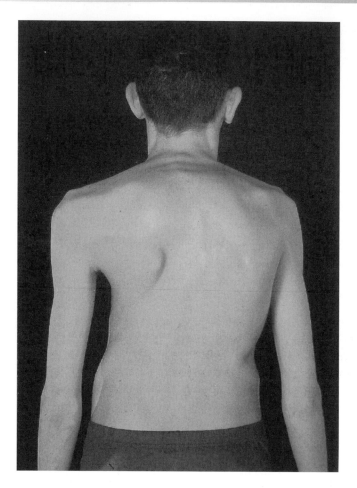

Figure 7 Lateral curvature of the spine or scoliosis.

Table 2 A brief classification of spinal deformities based upon the recommendations of the scolosis research society

1. Idiopathic	Scoliosis: Early onset (<5 years), Late onset (>5 years) Kyphosis: Scheurmann's Disease
2. Congenital	Bone deformities (failure of formation and segmentation) Spinal cord deformities (spina bifida and myelodysplasia)
3. Neuromuscular	Cerebral palsy, poliomyelitis, muscular dystrophies
4. Neurofibromatosis	
5. Mesenchymal disorders	Marfan's syndrome, Osteogenesis imperfecta
6. Traumatic	
7. Post infective	Pyogenic or tuberculous
8. Tumours	
9. Miscellanous	

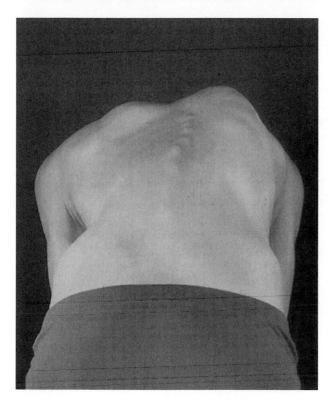

Figure 8 The rib hump on forward bending in structural scoliosis.

and whether part of the curve is correctable. Decompensation signs of the curve should be assessed by using the plumb line as well as looking at the gait and assessing the secondary curves (**Table 2**).

Measure the range of motion of the spine in flexion, extension, lateral flexion and rotation. The latter should be either sitting or by holding the pelvis when standing. Assess true spinal movement in forward flexion, for the hips could compensate. Straight leg raising test passive and active should be performed and this could be restricted due to nerve root irritation as in acute disc protrusion. Tight hamstrings with increased popliteal angles could be a feature of spondylolysis with low back pain.

Lower limbs

Standing examination includes the Trendelenburg test and the block test for limb length inequality.

Trendelenburg test

Failure of the abductor mechanism producing a positive trendelenburg test is due to instability at the fulcrum in DDH, failure of the lever arm as in a short or varus femoral neck or pseudoarthroses and failure of the power arm due to a neurological cause for weakness of the abductors. A delayed Trendelenburg test assesses the abductor fatigue on loading with time and is positive in acetabular dysplasia.

The Trendelenburg test is performed by asking the child to stand on each leg with both hips in extension and the non weight-bearing knee flexed. Normally standing on the unaffected side elevates the pelvis on the opposite side (**Figure 9**). A positive test is when the opposite side of the pelvis drops indicating failure of the abductor mechanism (**Figure 10**). The delayed Trendelenburg test is to make the child stand for 30 seconds to assess the abductors' fatigue as in acetabular dysplasia.

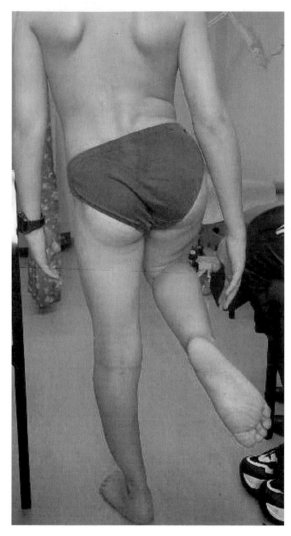

Figure 9 The pelvis being elevated when standing on the unaffected or normal side.

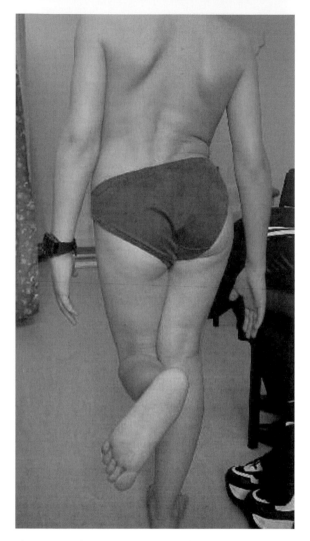

Figure 10 The positive Trendelenburg test due to Tom Smith arthritis of infancy.

Limb length discrepancy

Limb length discrepancy is assessed by the block test (**Figure 11**). Blocks are of different sizes and the child is made to stand with hips and knees extended and feet together with the shorter side on the blocks. The level of the PSIS, the highest point of the iliac crests and the ASIS can all be used as landmarks. True shortening can be measured this way only if there is no FFD at the hip or at the knee. If present the child should be measured in the supine position placing the normal leg in the same position as the affected side. The same rule holds good if associated adduction or abduction deformities are present. Adduction deformities produce apparent shortening of the limb and abduction deformities make the leg appear longer.

To determine whether shortening is above or below the knee, the Galeazzi test is done with the child lying supine and flexing both the knees at a right

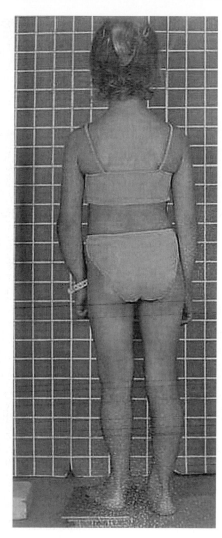

Figure 11 The block test to equalize limb lengths.

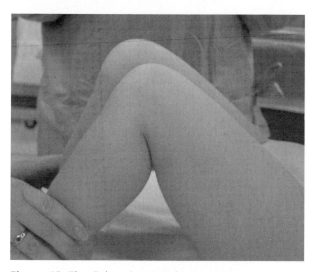

Figure 12 The Galeazzi test to demonstrate asymmetrical knee heights in a dislocated hip.

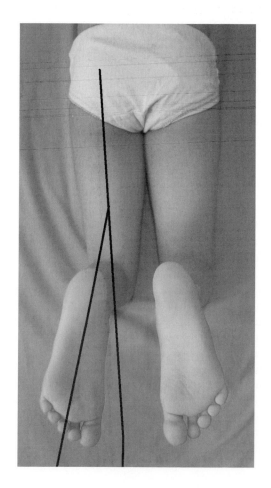

Figure 13 The prone examination to assess the thigh foot angle.

angle and the heels together. The mismatch in the knee heights when seen from the side will suggest whether the discrepancy is in the femur or tibia (**Figure 12**). The Bryant's test can then be used to reveal whether a femoral shortening if present is supra or infra trochanteric by palpating the relative positions of the tips of the trochanters and ASIS on either side using the thumbs on the ASIS, the middle finger on the tip of the greater trochanter and the index finger perpendicular to the couch.

Rotational profile

The foot progression angle and patellar progression angles seen on visual gait analysis will suggest intoeing or outoeing but not necessarily the segment for the cause. Remember muscular forces can also influence this, especially in a spastic gait. Prone examination is the best way to determine the site for the torsional anomalies. With the child prone and flexed at the knees the feet can be assessed for metatarsus varus or other deformities. The thigh foot angle reflects tibial torsion and is measured by drawing an imaginary line along the long axis of the femur and a line bisecting the foot in it's resting position. Normal value is 10-15 degrees of external rotation (**Figure 13**). Alternatively the trans-malleolar axis can be used in the sitting position by comparing the transcondylar axis of the tibia with the bimalleolar axis, which is usually about 20 degrees of external rotation.

Then examine the hip for the range of internal and external rotation and perform the Gage test, which determines the femoral anteversion. The leg is used as the lever and the axis of the tibia as a reference. The examiners' thumb is on the trochanter and the palm of the hand on the buttock. The angle created by the leg to the imaginary vertical line when the greater trochanter becomes most prominent on rotating the limb from maximum internal rotation to maximum external rotation, is the angle of anteversion of the femur. Femoral torsion is described when this is above 2 standard deviations to the normal. Therefore there will be excessive internal rotation in femoral torsion and restricted or absent internal rotation in retrotorsion of the hip as in congenital short femora. The femoral anteversion at birth is about 40 degrees, 20 degrees by the age of 9

and reaches the adult value of 16 by the age of 16 years.

Hip

General inspection on supine examination is for any scars from previous surgery or sinuses from infection. Any asymmetrical creases especially at the groin extending to the buttock may be associated with developmental dysplasia of the hip. The attitude of the limb should be assessed and whether there's any apparent limb length discrepancy. Any effusion in the joint produces a flexion, abduction and external rotation attitude of the limb as in an irritable hip. The limb appears longer with a fixed abduction deformity and the ipsilateral ASIS is at a lower level. In adduction deformities the limb appears shorter and the ipsilateral ASIS is at a higher level.

Palpate the bony landmarks around the hip for tenderness including the greater trochanter. Eliciting palpatory findings of the hip joint per se is difficult as it is deeply placed. The femoral head may be palpable in the groin in partially treated DDH or in dysplastic hips otherwise called the "lump sign". The femoral head is made more palpable with the limb held in external rotation. The greater trochanter may be broadened in Perthes Disease.

Before assessing range of motion of the hip joint , concealed deformities need to be revealed. The Thomas test is done to reveal a fixed flexion deformity at the hip (**Figure 14**). This is concealed by an exaggerated lumbar lordosis. The contralateral hip is flexed to its maximum and held there by the child holding the knee, whilst the examiner confirms flattening of the lumbar lordosis using the palm of his hand. The child is then asked to gently extend the other leg. The angle created by the thigh segment with the couch is the angle of the fixed flexion deformity. Then the range of flexion in this hip is determined the manoeuvre repeated on the opposite side. The alternative to this test is Stahelis' prone hip extension test where the child is stabilised at the bottom of the couch in prone position with both limbs free and supported and then visually flattening the lordosis by flexing both hips. The hip is then extended and when the buttock starts to rise, the

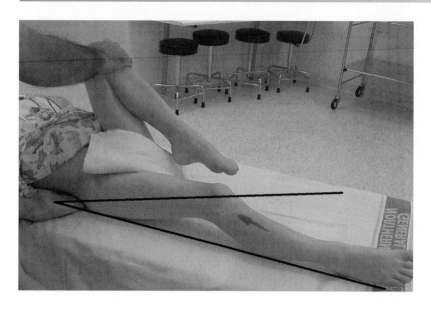

Figure 14 The Thomas test to reveal the fixed flexion deformity at the hip.

angle created by the thigh to the lumbosacral spine is the amount of fixed flexion deformity at the hip.

Coronal plane movement is assessed after stabilizing the pelvis and confirming that the pelvis is square. Maximum abduction of the unaffected side is a good method of locking the pelvis. When deformities exist in this plane the pelvis is squared and the further range of motion in that plane is assessed.

Rotation of the hip is best assessed with the hips in extension and the child prone. Rotation with the hip in 90 degrees of flexion can be assessed, but is of less significance.

In irritable hip conditions, the earliest movement lost is adduction in flexion and normally there should be at least 20 degrees in this position.

Telescoping test is positive in late presentation of dislocated hips or due to old septic arthritis of infancy (Tom Smith arthritis). This is elicited with the hip and knee flexed and with the pelvis stabilized, the thigh is loaded downwards and released, feeling the femoral head or trochanter moving vertically.

When examining neonates for DDH, the Ortolani test is to elicit the sign of entry of the hip from the dislocated position followed by exit to it's dislocated position. The test is done with the child relaxed on the couch with one hand stabilizing the pelvis and the other flexing the knee fully and flexing the hip to 90 degrees. The thumb is on the inside with the other three fingers on the trochanter. As the hip is abducted a palpable and audible "clunk" is a positive test for reduction and when the opposite manoeuvre is done the clunk of exit is recorded as displacement of the hip. The Barlow's test is a provocative test for instability, elicited the same way but demonstrating the clunk of exit from the acetabular rim by gently pushing with the thumb on the adducted hip. Dynamic and static ultrasound examination is the gold standard in assessing instability or dysplasia and monitoring progress of treatment up to the age of 6 months. The later classic signs in DDH are those of asymmetrical thigh folds, limitation of abduction and relative shortening of the femur with the knees in flexion (positive Galleazzi sign). The Ortolani and Barlow's tests are not useful after the age of 6 months. A plain AP radiograph of the hips after the age of 3-6 months can be used to diagnose DDH.

Children with Perthes Disease lose abduction in flexion quite early. They also show features of irritability at the hip and gradually also lack internal rotation. When the hip is flexed the knee deviates towards the ipsilateral shoulder. This is a good clinical sign for early femoral head deformity. Spasm can produce deformities at the hip and if complicated with chondrolysis can become fixed. Serial radiographs AP and frog leg lateral views will show the different evolutionary stages in the process of healing from avascular necrosis with the crescent sign, stage of fragmentation or revascularisation and healing.

Children with a slipped capital femoral epiphysis have decreased abduction, internal rotation and flexion, whereas they gain adduction, external rotation and extension. Flexing the hip causes the knee to deviate towards the ipsilateral shoulder as in Perthes Disease. The presence of a fixed flexion deformity as well, suggests that the hip is developing chondrolysis. An outoeing gait is one presentation especially in the chronic slips. A frog leg lateral view of the hips will demonstrate the extent of the slip and also show the early slip, which could be missed in the AP film. The percentage of slip can also be measured on this view.

Knee

Inspect the knee for any swelling. Fullness of the parapatellar fossae suggests a small effusion and a horseshoe swelling of the suprapatellar fossa larger effusions (**Figure 15**). Generalised swelling is seen in inflammatory synovitis. Localised swellings could result from bursae or bony lumps such as the tibial tuberosity in Osgood-Schlatter's Disease. Any colour change with redness and signs of inflammation should be noted. The semimembranous bursa is commonly seen on the posteromedial aspect of the knee. Coronal plane deformities of genu valgum or genu varum should be assessed standing. Up to the age of 2 years, a moderate degree of genu varum is normal. This then develops into excessive valgus by the age of three and normalizes to about 7 degrees of valgus by the age of 5-7 years.

The knee is palpated to elicit tenderness at the joint lines for the menisci and bony landmarks (e.g. tibial tuberosity) as well as the patellar undersurface for chondromalacia. For smaller effusions, the bulge test can elicit fluid in the joint and for moderate effusions the patellar tap can be done after squeezing the suprapatellar pouch (**Figure 16**). A tense haemarthrosis does not have a positive patellar tap.

Active range of motion is best elicited before passive movements. Determine whether there is any fixed flexion deformity at the knee as is seen in discoid menisci. Compare the movements of the good knee

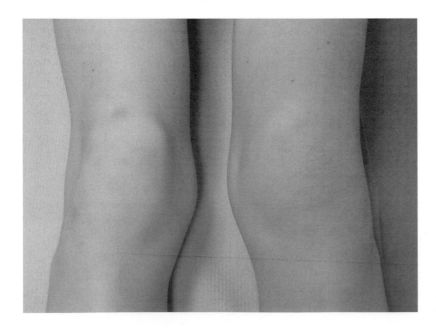

Figure 15 The fullness of the parapatellar fossae and the suprapatellar pouch in a large effusion.

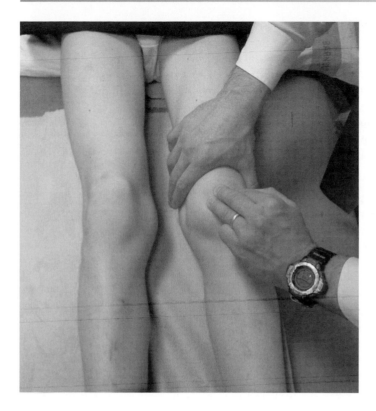

Figure 16 Demonstration of the patellar tap.

with the affected one, both in flexion and extension. Hyperextension at the knee is recorded as well as symmetry and any associated features of benign hypermobility.

Patellar position whether high (alta) or low (baja) is noted. Patellar tracking in the sitting position with the legs free can demonstrate lateral squinting and tilting, habitual dislocation or subluxation. The patellar apprehension test is elicited by attempting to push the patella laterally in an extended position and then flexing the knee. The child will resist this movement due to discomfort and apprehension if instability exists. Patellofemoral crepitus can be elicited on moving the knee and applying patellofemoral compression against the femoral trochlea. Ligamentous stability should be tested next. Lachman's test with the knee in 10-20 degrees of flexion looks for abnormal movement in the anteroposterior plane and assesses anterior cruciate deficiency as seen in congenital short femur or lon-

gitudinal deficiencies of the lower limbs as well as in the older child who sustains a tear of the ACL. Posterior sag of the knee can be assessed with the knee held at a right angle to the couch demonstrating posterior cruciate deficiency as in some severe longitudinal congenital deficiencies. The collateral ligaments are tested with the knee in extension and in 30 degrees of flexion with varus and valgus force. Ligamentous laxity is associated with many skeletal dysplasias and therefore needs to be recorded.

Foot and ankle

Examine the feet standing, walking and at rest. On standing the heel is in slight valgus to the long axis of the calf due to subtalar mobility. The arch may be flat (pes planus), normal or high as in pes cavus. Callosities on the sole of the feet tell you the weight bearing pattern and also the soles of the shoes and their uppers. Neuropathic ulcers may be seen in spina bifida and in sensory neuropathic conditions.

Deformities of the toes need to be noted. Curly lesser toes, overriding 2nd toes, overriding 5th toes, hammer and mallet toes are some of the common deformities. Clawing of the toes warrants an examination of the spine to exclude spinal dysraphism, as well as investigations for other conditions like hereditary sensorimotor neuropathies or Friedreich's Ataxia. Metatarsus adductus or varus may be noted and could be part of a serpentine or skew foot or a residual clubfoot deformity.

The foot should be palpated over all bony landmarks. Tenderness over the calcaneum could reflect calcaneal apophysitis (Sever's Disease). Tenderness around the second metatarso-phalangeal joint might reflect Freiberg's Disease. When assessing mobility of the foot, deformities need to be noted. Ankle range of motion in plantarflexion and dorsiflexion, subtalar movement in eversion and inversion and midfoot movement in all planes needs to be recorded. Any deformity should be assessed as being fixed or correctable, partially or completely. Reduced subtalar movement as in spasmodic peroneal flatfoot is seen in tarsal coalitions in adolescents and subtalar irritability in seronagative inflammatory conditions.

Flatfeet are associated with dropped medial longitudinal arches on standing and valgus heels. When the child is made to stand tiptoes they recreate the arch and the heel goes into neutral or varus when there is no underlying abnormality. The same reconstitution of flexible flatfeet can be seen on dorsiflexing the big toe and on standing with external rotation of the tibia. Flexible flatfeet with tight heelcords need to be identified, as they require treatment. Rigid flatfeet can be either of the type seen in spasmodic peroneal flatfeet of any cause or the rockerbottom type seen in congenital vertical talus or in association with other conditions or syndromes such as spina bifida, and Arthrogyposis multiplex congenita.

Pes cavus can result from plantaris deformities of the forefoot, equinocavus or in association with calcaneocavus. Fixed pronation deformities of the forefoot seen in peroneal muscular atrophy can produce a varus posture of the heel on standing. This may be fully correctable. The Coleman block test can be used to elicit this. The child is asked to stand on a block, which supports the heel and lateral border of the foot allowing the first metatarsal to drop. The heel should correct to a neutral or valgus position if the hindfoot deformity is mobile suggesting that the heel varus is due to a fixed pronation deformity of the forefoot.

Examination of the muscles around the foot and ankle is important and muscle strength should be graded as per MRC grading. The foot deformities can be due to varied aetiological causes and may be structural as in CTEV, muscular as in Duchenne muscular dystrophy, peripheral nerve disorders as in peroneal muscular atrophy, lower nerve roots as in spinal dysraphism or due to upper motor neurone disorders as in cerebral palsy

Upper limbs

Shoulder

Observe the contour of the shoulder from the front, back and the side. A high scapula as in Sprengel's shoulder can be seen even from the front. The scapula may be hypoplastic and wider sideways. This could be in association with Klippel-Feil Syndrome with shortening and webbing of the neck and a low posterior hairline. Webbing of the neck may also be seen in Turner's Syndrome. Abnormalities of the axillary pectoral folds could be due to absence of the sternal part of the pectoralis major as in Poland's Syndrome. Children with hereditary multiple exostoses often have lumps around the shoulder.

Palpation of the shoulder joint and upper humerus should be done for tenderness and lumps. Absent clavicles may be seen in cleidocranial dysostoses and defects of the clavicle may be palpable in pseudoarthroses of the clavicle.

Assess the range of motion of the shoulder joint active first and then passive. The glenohumeral movement is examined by stabilising the scapula and then the scapulothoracic movements without any restriction of the scapula. Children can be asked to clap their hands in forward flexion or over their heads if not co-operative.

Stability of the shoulder is assessed next by stressing the humeral head forwards and backwards and by the sulcus test by pulling on the arm downwards. Multidirectional instability can be demonstrated in the atraumatic groups with bilateral signs and in association with ligamentous laxity. The apprehension test for anterior shoulder instability is performed by attempting to abduct and externally rotate the shoulder. The child resists in a positive test. Quite often the child can demonstrate the clunk or instability of the shoulder themselves. It is worthwhile getting the child to elicit this to see the shoulder action and the direction of instability.

Elbow

The elbow is relatively an easy joint to examine in a child. Swelling and deformities are well seen. In full extension the carrying angle can be assessed and is normally 10-15 degrees being more in females. Comparison of the unaffected side gives quantification of any deformity. A reduced carrying angle is seen in malunited supracondylar fractures and when severe produces the gunstock deformity which looks quite ugly when seen from the back or when the child walks. An increased carrying angle is noted in Turner's Syndrome.

Palpation of bony landmarks around the elbow is undertaken in a fixed manner. The normal triangular relationship of the epicondyles and tip of the olecranon with the elbow in flexion and the linear relationship with the elbow in extension give clues to assess malunion of the distal humerus. Palpation of the radial head and the assessment of rotation of the forearm may reveal abnormalities of the relationship of the radial head with the capitellum as in missed Monteggia fractures or congenital dislocation.

Movements of the elbow joint should be recorded and compared to the normal side. Hyperextension can be noted in association with laxity or in malunited supracondylar fractures. With the elbow in flexion at right angles forearm rotation is assessed. This might be restricted or completely absent in radio-ulnar synostoses. Examination of shoulder rotation can be used to evaluate varus malunion in supracondylar fractures producing increased internal rotation.

Wrist and hand

The wrist can be assessed for swellings such as ganglia classically on the dorsum or on the radio-volar aspect. Prominence of the lower end of ulna with radial and volar deviation of the wrist is seen in a Madelung deformity which may be bilateral in the familial condition or unilateral if acquired as in posttraumatic physeal arrest of the distal radius. The wrist can be easily assessed for tenderness, swellings, synovial thickening and any increase in warmth. Movements are assessed and also ligamentous laxity as seen with hypermobility when the thumb is able to approximate the volar aspect of the wrist.

Generalised systemic disorders can be detected by clubbing or cyanosis of the fingers. Common finger deformities such as the Kirner deformity of the little finger, clinodactyly, camptodactyly, syndactyly and polydactyly are easily seen. Arachnodactyly can be a clue for Marfan's Syndrome. Hypoplasia of the upper limb and hand can be appreciated when compared to the normal side.

Finger movements are also a good indication of ligamentous laxity with hyperextension at the MCP joints. Joint ranges need to be assessed. Neurological examination is important in posttraumatic sequelae when associated with neurovascular injuries. Abnormalities of sensation may be difficult to assess in the younger child. Examining the sweat pattern of the hand is an indication of sensory loss. Examining for individual peripheral nerves and documentation of recovery pattern helps in the follow-up. Any ischaemic sequelae of compartment syndrome needs to be identified and differentiated from neurological injury. Asking the child to spread the fingers and demonstrate a "five", adduct the fingers with the thumb in hand to show a "four", making a fist and showing the letter "o" with the thumb and index finger reliably assesses the motor supply of the hand. Strength can be assessed by asking the child to grasp your hand. Test also the pinch and the hook functions.

Neuromuscular Examination

Cerebral palsy

The sequence of examination should be in one's own style and has to be modified depending on the age of the child, and whether they can stand and walk or not. Children younger than 5 years of age can be examined on their mother's lap to start with. The child who can stand and walk can be assessed standing followed by observational gait analysis, sitting and then supine. The child who cannot walk should be first assessed in the wheelchair followed by sitting and finally supine. Brief upper limb examination, head and neck control and associated defects need to be assessed. Look for athetoid movements or any abnormal dystonic posturing or other abnormal involuntary movements.

Lower limb assessment: Range of movements should be recorded methodically and muscle testing as per MRC grading if possible. Leg lengths should be measured with the patient supine with appropriate positioning depending on pelvic obliquity and contractures. Measurement of the true leg length is important in these children.

Hip: The Thomas test is used to elicit the fixed flexion deformity at each hip and further range of motion is measured. Staheli's prone hip extension test is a worthwhile alternative test as it's more accurate in cerebral palsy children. In the same position, hip rotations can also be assessed. The Gage test will determine the angle of femoral anteversion and femoral torsion is commonly associated with this neuromuscular condition. The prone rectus femoris test demonstrates a tight rectus when the buttock elevates as the knee is rapidly flexed. Hip abduction and adduction should be examined with the hips in extension and in flexion.

Knee: Spasticity and contracture of the hamstrings can be reliably measured by straight leg raising and assessing the popliteal angle. The hip is flexed to 90 degrees and then the knee is extended from the flexed position. The angle created by the front of the leg to the front of the thigh is the popliteal angle (**Figure 17**). Normal values are less than 20 degrees. Any fixed flexion contracture at the knee should be assessed by extending the limb maximally and if present will be due to posterior capsular contracture. Quadriceps strength and spasticity can be assessed next. Phelp's gracilis test is done with the

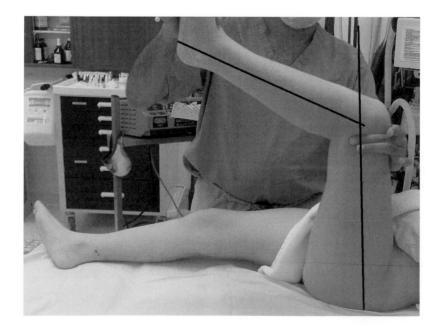

Figure 17 The popliteal angle used to assess tight hamstrings.

patient prone, knees flexed and hips abducted. If the hip adducts on extending the knee, gracilis spasm or contracture are confirmed.

Foot and ankle: The range of motion at the ankle is recorded. The Silverskiold test differentiates gastrocnemius contracture from that of the soleus. If dorsiflexion of the foot is greater when the knee is flexed than when it's extended, then the gastrocnemius is implicated as the main site of contracture. If there is no change then contracture of both muscles is present. Varus of the foot could be due to a spastic tibialis posterior muscle at the hindfoot or the tibialis anterior at the midfoot or both. It could be a dynamic deformity more appreciable when the child walks or a fixed deformity. Tibial torsion needs to be assessed in the sitting position using imaginary lines between the proximal condyles and the distal transmalleolar axis. Alternatively on prone examination the thigh-foot angle gives an idea about tibial torsion.

Other paralytic conditions

Knowledge of examining individual muscle groups and for nerve roots is essential in assessing children with paralytic conditions like Poliomyelitis or Spina bifida disorders. Sensory dermatomal distribution and knowledge of autonomic systems supplying the bowel and bladder is essential.

Ober's test is used to assess the tightness of the iliotibial band and any abduction contracture at the hip. The test is performed by asking the child to lie on the side opposite to the one being tested. The uninvolved hip and knee are maximally flexed to flatten the lumbar spine. The hip to be tested is then flexed to 90 degrees with the knee flexed and then fully abducted. The hip is then brought into full hyperextension and allowed to adduct maximally. The angle that the thigh makes with a horizontal line parallel to the table is the degree of contracture at the hip. The iliotibial band when tight produces deformities at the knee of flexion, external rotation and valgus (the triple deformity). Gradual posterior subluxation and secondary deformities of equinus at the ankle, pelvic obliquity, scoliosis and limb length discrepancy may develop.

Further reading

Apley AG, Solomon L. *Apley's System of Orthopaedics and Fractures, Seventh Edition*. Butterworth Heinemann, Oxford: 1993.

Benson MKD, Fixsen JA, Macnicol MF. *Children's Orthopaedics and Fractures, First Edition*, Churchill Livingstone, London: 1994.

Bleck EE. Orthopaedic Management in Cerebral Palsy - *Clinics in Developmental Medicine* No. 99/100, MacKeith Press, Philadelphia: 1987.

Broughton NS. *Paediatric Orthopaedics*, W.B. Saunders, Philadelphia 1996.

Gage JR. Gait analysis in Cerebral Palsy - *Clinics in Developmental Medicine* No. 121, MacKeith Press, Oxford: 1991.

Tachdjian MO. *Pediatric Orthopedics, First Edition*, WB Saunders, Philadelphia: 1990.

12

Examination of the Spine in Childhood

N Chiverton & R A Dickson

Introduction

Children are referred to spinal clinics usually as a result of a visible deformity but sometimes with pain. Some will come via their general practitioner but many come via general orthopaedic surgeons with an interest in children's' orthopaedic disorders or from paediatricians or paediatric neurologists who look after the many childhood conditions that can be associated with a spinal deformity. Interestingly, with universal use of antenatal ultrasound some deformities such as congenital hemivertebrae, can lead to referrals early in utero.

The spectrum of conditions which the children's spinal surgeon may expect to see includes spinal infection, discitis, trauma, tumours, spondylolysis and spondylisthesis, the adolescent disc syndrome, as well as spinal deformities. As with children's hip problems it is important to consider the age of the child. For example pyogenic spinal infection can occur throughout childhood whereas TB generally occurs under the age of three. Discitis generally occurs between the ages of three and eight while scoliosis has two principal ages of onset, in infancy and in early adolescence. Kyphosis tends to present towards the end of adolescence.

Red flags in the history would include night pain (bone destructive lesion until proven otherwise) and continuous rather than episodic pain (again suggestive of tumour). If tumour is suspected under the age of six, three-quarters are malignant whereas over the age of six, less than a third. Neck trauma is more often in the upper cervical spine unlike the adult counterpart. Watch out for an atypical scoliosis (left thoracic curve, progressive curve in a boy, painful or stiff curve, curve in association with headache) as a syrinx, which is sometimes malignant, must be excluded. Spinal tenderness is only really a feature of spinal infection or fresh fracture which makes the diagnostic triad of fever, back pain and tenderness, typical of spinal infection, easy to recognise. However, spinal infection is notorious for delay in diagnosis and wrong diagnosis before the correct one is made. Delay in diagnosis is also common with discitis and the adolescent disc syndrome, which with longish natural histories, tends to strain patient/family doctor relationships. Don't forget to ask questions about the child's general health. Is the appetite good and is weight being gained or is there evidence of failure to thrive? Any concerns here should raise the possibility of infection or tumour?

Specific Conditions and their Related Symptoms

Scoliosis

The great majority will be idiopathic and there are two ages of onset, infancy and adolescence. In the latter, intermittent fatigue discomfort over the rib hump is common and anything more intrusive needs an MRI scan or bone scan to exclude syrinx or tumour. Respiratory problems only occur with infantile progressive scoliosis when the chest wall is deformed at the same time as the alveoli reduplicate and therefore a respiratory assessment may be crucial in early onset scoliosis.

In assessing a spinal deformity in infants it is important to ask the child's birth weight, whether there were any obstetric complications, and whether the child is going through milestones at a natural rate. Any problems here may suggest a likelihood of progression. Ask about a family history as scoliosis, kyphosis and spondylolisthesis are all familial. In assessing the older child and adolescent the history part of the consultation is all-important. How old the child is biologically indicates the potential for future progression. When was the first period as peak adolescent growth velocity occurs just beyond this time? Alternatively, if the child has stopped growing the risk of future progression is minimal. As no non-operative treatment alters natural history for patients with late onset idiopathic scoliosis, it is important to find out if the deformity is acceptable to the patient and family because unacceptability is the only indication for surgical treatment. Unacceptability means having sufficient concern about spinal shape to agree to major spinal surgery not without significant risks. This is a very subjective and individualistic matter. All one can do is to observe the deformity over many years of growth, when regular meetings with the patient and family give plenty of time to enquire about the impact of the deformity and whether the family are inclining towards a surgical solution. The role of the surgeon in the history taking part of the consultation is to help the family to make the right decision. Late onset idiopathic scoliosis is not a matter of organic ill-health or physical spinal dysfunction (teenage girls with scoliosis can just as well be nurses and P.E. teachers as anything else), it is solely a matter of appearance.

Kyphosis

There are two types of idiopathic kyphosis:

- Type 1, lower thoracic Scheuermann's Disease
- Type 2, thoraco-lumbar Scheuermann's Disease sometimes referred to as Apprentice's spine.

The former presents in the last two years of adolescent growth and the latter in the late teens and early twenties. Either deformity or pain is complained of, or both. Again, the pain should be mechanical and intermittent and not suggestive of any bone destructive lesion. Neurological symptoms are only complained of in very extreme degrees of kyphosis.

Idiopathic kyphosis (Scheuermann's Disease) is eminently treatable conservatively by extension bracing and as surgery is perhaps more complex and less rewarding than surgery for idiopathic scoliosis the surgeon should counsel strongly about the need for bracing and to try to maintain compliance. Thus the history part of the consultation is not merely a matter of asking questions and gathering information but constitutes an important dialogue with the patient and family with the surgeon often adopting a pro-active rather than a reactive role.

Notwithstanding, a severe roundback deformity in a shape-conscious individual can be just as devastating, if not more so, than a comparable scoliotic deformity.

Spondylolysis / Spondylolisthesis

This is probably the commonest cause of low back pain in childhood and lyses have a surprisingly high prevalence rate of 3% in three year olds and 10% in adolescents to the point where the presence

of such a lesion is not considered necessarily to be a risk factor for back pain. Any pain that does result should be associated with repetitive bending and twisting episodes such as with gymnasts, trampolinists and fast bowlers as well as ballet dancers, and reciprocally should settle with cessation of exercise. Neurological symptoms are very uncommon except with lytic spondylolistheses when the callus surrounding the lysis (effectively a fracture non-union) may irritate the locally exiting nerve root (L5 for an L5/S1 spondylolisthesis). Therefore it is necessary to enquire into sporting and recreational activities.

Other conditions

Although we stressed the importance of night pain in association with tumour, in fact back pain is only present in about a third with limp and leg weakness occurring in the majority. With osteoblastoma and its smaller counterpart osteoid osteoma pain is typically at the thoraco-lumbar junction and relieved by non-steroidal anti-inflammatory drugs. Delay in diagnosis and chronicity can produce psychological dysfunction.

The child with cerebral palsy or one of the severe neuromuscular conditions of childhood such as congenital muscular dystrophy or spinal muscular atrophy will almost certainly have been seen already by a paediatric neurologist but a history of normal neurological development and leg function with a recent change to weakness or limp, would raise concerns about tumour.

Examination

As with all musculoskeletal parts examination comprises inspection, palpation, range of motion, and special tests.

Children are not referred with a letter "Dear Mr so and so ? back please" but rather with more specific instructions such as "I think this young lady has developed a spinal deformity" or "this boy of seven has recently complained of low back pain" and thus not only is the history targeted but so is the physical examination.

Examination of the infant or very young child

It is useful to have the baby sitting on mother's knee with nothing on but a nappy facing mother. On first inspection gain a general impression of the child as to its size. Is it alert, turning round to look at you all the time? Does it have head and trunk control? Does the child look well or does it look undernourished? Does it look miserable and possibly in pain, which might suggest the possibility of infection or tumour? The spine should be carefully palpated but it is more often not possible to localise the pathology on examination. Then, looking from above and from the back note the presence of any spinal deformity with its associated rotational prominence on the convex side. Record the site and direction of the curve and note if it is a single or double curve (right thoracic curves in girls and double structural curves have more significant progression potential). From above note the shape of the head as plagiocephaly is commonly associated with infantile scoliosis. Look for plagiothorax and plagiocephaly as well as a bat ear, wry neck and relatively adducted hip, again all moulding features of infantile scoliosis. For the child referred with a wry neck only, palpate the sternomastoids for tightness particularly at the sterno-clavicular junction. A wry neck without sternomastoid tightness might suggest an underlying congenital cervico-thoracic scoliosis. Observe for the short neck and low hair-line of the Klippel-Feil Syndrome and observe the heights of the scapulae for the associated Sprengel's deformity.

It is difficult to perform a neurological examination in someone of this age but look and see if the child is kicking and using all muscle groups in the lower extremities and does the child crawl or attempt to stand or walk appropriate for its age. A walking child can be more formally assessed neurologically. Take the opportunity of checking leg lengths and hip range of motion.

Upper motor neurone features in the legs possibly in association with absent or asymmetric abdominal reflexes are strongly suggestive of tumour, particularly in association with a mild but stiff or painful scoliosis.

In addition to a low birth weight floppy hypotonic baby, curve rigidity is also an adverse prognostic factor and this is best assessed by lying the child convex side down over your knee and letting the head and pelvis sag. Over-correction in this position implies good flexibility. Observe for any lower extremity wasting, foot deformity, or spinal dysraphism (hairy patch, dimple, port wine stain, naevus, in the midline, which might suggest the presence of a congenital anomaly). The back of the nappy will have to be pulled down for these features to be seen.

Virtually diagnostic is the young child with a rigid hyperlordotic and painful lumbar spine who does not have a fever and is not systemically unwell. This is a non-infective discitis, which may be an autoimmune condition.

It is unusual for the severe neuromuscular conditions of childhood to be associated with a scoliosis in this age group, rather there is a floppy overall hyperkyphosis in the very young.

Examination of the older child or adolescent

Undressing down to underpants, or bra and pants, is essential. The standard examination procedure for the scoliosis patient is to inspect the back standing and leaning forward when the rotational prominence is maximised. Multiple curve patterns are more common than single curves and therefore, particularly on forward bending, look out for a lower left loin prominence in the patient who appears to have a single right thoracic curve. In the erect position note the height of the shoulders. For a right thoracic curve the left shoulder is lower but if it is higher (the signe d'epaule) then this indicates the presence of an upper left thoracic curve confirming a double thoracic curve pattern. If this is associated with a left loin prominence then a triple curve pattern is present and is not uncommon. In the erect position also assess flexibility with maximum side bending. Assess flexibility also by trying to compress the rib prominence. Suspend a plumb line from the vertebra prominens which should cut the natal cleft but if it lies to side of the convexity of the major curve then the spine is said to be "decompensated". Look for the cutaneous stigmata of spinal dysraphism which must be midline. Look also for the cutaneous manifestations of Von Reckling-hausen's Disease particularly café-au-lait spots and look in the axillae for freckling. Look for the excessive scarring, particularly of the knees, with Ehlers-Danlos Syndrome. On inspection from the front with a thoracic curve the chest wall will be more prominent on the concave side and indeed apparent breast asymmetry may be a reason for initial presentation. Observe also the waist asymmetry with a thoraco-lumbar or lumbar curve which patients often find as distressing as a rib hump.

Then examine the patient supine and put the hips and knees through a natural range of motion. Straight leg raising should not be impaired with idiopathic scoliosis and if there is evidence of hamstring tightness that raises the possibility of spinal tumour or spondylolisthesis. Neurological examination should be carried out and remember to assess the abdominal reflexes as absence or asymmetry indicates the presence of a syrinx. Inspect the lower extremities and measure leg lengths if inspection suggests inequality. Inequality of a centimetre or less may not be abnormal but if there is associated global reduction in size this would indicate the possibility of spinal dysraphysm and such a limb would tend to be hyporeflexic. Reduction in pain and temperature but a normal appreciation of touch indicates the presence of "suspended" disassociated sensory loss of a syrinx or intramedullary tumour.

When examining the kyphosis patient note whether the kyphosis is in the mid-lower thoracic spine for typical type 1 Scheuermann's Disease. In type 2 Scheuermann's Disease the kyphosis is less obvious and at the thoraco-lumbar or upper lumbar region. For type 1 Scheuermann's Disease, on forward bending, the kyphosis will be seen to have a definite apex which will be uncorrectable either by manual compression or thoracic hyperextension. By contrast, the postural roundback deformity is a gentle kyphosis, which is fully correctable. In the erect position observe the region of compensatory lumbar hyperlordosis where there is more often than not an appreciable degree of idiopathic scoliosis confirmed on forward bending by the presence of a loin hump. Straight leg raising is characteristically reduced with Scheuermann's Disease indicative of hamstring tightness. Perform a neurological examination.

When examining children with neuromuscular scolioses remember that there are two fundamental curve types – "balanced curves" going down to a square pelvis and "unbalanced curves" going down to a tilted pelvis. The latter tend to be long and C-shaped and such patients may spend some or all of their time in a wheelchair. Examination of the balanced curve is no different from that of idiopathic curves. These will be walkers so note their gait pattern for the broadly based gait of Friedreich's Ataxia or the high stepping gait with cavo-varus feet typical of the peripheral neuropathies. It is important also to observe the gait pattern in those that are still walkers because complex lumbo-pelvic twisting and bending is essential for locomotion and will be abolished by a spinal fusion which in turn may render a walker wheelchair bound.

The sitting patient can be examined in the wheelchair but if cooperation is possible it is better to sit them on the edge of an examination couch and inspect from the back. The typical long thoraco-lumbar curve down to an oblique pelvis will be seen and by suspending the child under the arms. A considerable flexibility is the rule rather than the exception. Does the child have head control and, importantly, does the child have sitting stability. This is assessed by raising the arms so that the hands are free of the examination couch and if the spine collapses, then sitting stability has been lost. Examine if the child can prop themselves up using their arms or whether sitting stability has been lost because of lack of central neuromuscular control which is crucial as sitting stability cannot be restored in the latter situation by surgical instrumentation and correction of the curve. Try and assess overall mental development in the cerebral palsy patient and try and formulate some opinion about whether the child has sufficient understanding of the situation to be co-operative and compliant to go through a difficult operative schedule.

Pelvic obliquity and its assessment by examination is commonly poorly understood and may be a concern for FRCS Orth candidates but it is straightforward. There are three types:

1. Suprapelvic

2. Transpelvic

3. Infrapelvic

Suprapelvic pelvic obliquity is caused by a collapsing neuromuscular scoliosis. Transpelvic pelvic obliquity is caused by unequal spasm in the iliopsoas muscles, the only ones to cross the pelvis from spine to lower extremity. For practical purposes this will only be encountered in cerebral palsy type individuals. Infrapelvic pelvic obliquity is caused by a leg length inequality either real or apparent from a hip contracture. Transpelvic pelvic obliquity may be correctable or fixed, in the latter when examining leg length inequality in a supine patient the pelvis cannot be put square to the trunk

Start the examination of the low back patient again in the erect position. The back is first inspected. Some flattening of the lumbar lordosis accompanies any painful low back condition, when combined with a mild lumbar scoliosis there is an association with the adolescent disc syndrome (disc protrusion/prolapse). A lumbo-sacral kyphosis indicates the presence of a dysplastic spondylolisthesis which, if accompanied by some degree of lumbar scoliosis and a thoraco-lumbar hyperlordosis above is commensurate with the adolescent crisis with the L5 vertebra rolling around precariously on top of the sacrum. Inspection from the front may reveal an abdominal skin crease in association with a dysplastic spondylolisthesis which is in effect compressed abdominal wall well in front of a lumbo-sacral kyphosis.

Flexion is often markedly reduced with the adolescent disc syndrome and impossible with dysplastic spondylolisthesis, any movements occurring at the hip joints. Flexion is best recorded in fractions of normal or perhaps measurement of fingertip to ground distance. It is important to watch the lumbar spine and see if the normal lordosis reverses and judge subjectively whether movements are occurring in the spine, at the hip joints, or both. The Schober Test (mark the lumbar spine at the level of the dimples of Venus and again 10 cms higher up and measure by how much they diverge on flexion) can be used if an accurate quantatative assessment is required. A step may be palpable with a lytic spondylolisthesis and this is at the level above the slip (i.e. the L4/5 spinous process level for an L5/S1 spondylolisthesis because the back of L5 is left behind due to the gap in the pars interarticularis). With bone destructive pathologies, there may be no abnormalities on inspection and palpation at all but with spinal infection there is often local tenderness to percussion.

On examination, supine straight leg raising is often markedly reduced in spondylolisthesis and may be absolutely nil or indeed negative with an inability to lie supine with extended hips and knees. A careful neurological examination is important looking in particular for long tract signs, signs of an intramedullary lesion and abdominal reflex abnormality.

Index